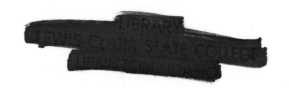

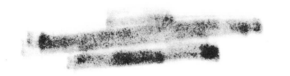

UNDERSTANDING
THE HUMAN BODY

For Churchill Livingstone:

Senior Commissioning Editor: Sarena Wolfaard
Project Development Manager: Mairi McCubbin
Project Manager: Gail Wright
Senior Designer: Judith Wright
Illustration Manager: Bruce Hogarth

UNDERSTANDING THE HUMAN BODY

Biological Perspectives for Healthcare

Helen Godfrey BSc(Hons) PhD RN SCM

Principal Lecturer, Faculty of Health and Social Care,
University of the West of England, Bristol, UK

Illustrations by
Graeme Chambers BA(Hons)
Medical Artist

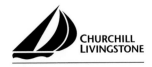

CHURCHILL
LIVINGSTONE

Edinburgh London New York Oxford Philadelphia St Louis Sydney Toronto 2004

CHURCHILL LIVINGSTONE
An imprint of Elsevier Limited

First published 2004

ISBN 0 443 07320 1

British Library Cataloguing in Publication Data
A catalogue record for this book is available from the British Library

Library of Congress Cataloging in Publication Data
A catalog record for this book is available from the Library of Congress

Notice
Medical knowledge is constantly changing. Standard safety precautions must be followed, but as new research and clinical experience broaden our knowledge, changes in treatment and drug therapy may become necessary or appropriate. Readers are advised to check the most current product information provided by the manufacturer of each drug to be administered to verify the recommended dose, the method and duration of administration, and contraindications. It is the responsibility of the practitioner, relying on experience and knowledge of the patient, to determine dosages and the best treatment for each individual patient. Neither the Publisher nor the author assumes any liability for any injury and/or damage to persons or property arising from this publication.

The Publisher

The Publisher's policy is to use paper manufactured from sustainable forests

Printed in China

Contents

Preface

'This book is all about what it is to be human from a biological perspective. It is intended to capture the imagination of anyone who wants to make sense of human bodies. The main aim has been to produce a book that is enjoyable to look at and, I hope, to read. I would like readers to be captivated and surprised by some of the amazing abilities and achievements of our bodies that are explored within these chapters. Rather than providing lots of detail and describing the human body as a machine, I have tried to give readers an insight into some of the really important and universal experiences, such as growing older, feeling stressed and being in pain. Unravelling the mysteries of sleep, explaining how genes shape our lives and describing the growth of an embryo from a single cell are just a few of the stories told here.

This book takes a rather unusual approach to helping readers to begin to understand what it means to be human. An essential difference from more traditional texts is that the reader does not have to read through huge amounts of detail, with the risk of giving up, but can immediately start to find out what makes us who we are. The reader will discover how to promote sleep, appreciate the important preventative factors in osteoporosis, and understand how aspirin helps to protect against coronary heart disease and how nutritional programming in fetuses and babies influences long-term health.

Despite the innovative style, the really important biological concepts and principles have been included and lots of contemporary references provided. I hope you enjoy the book and are inspired to discover more about the fundamentals of being human!

I would like to thank the many students, colleagues, friends and family members who have encouraged me to write this book and have often given me ideas and inspiration without realizing it.'

Bristol 2004   Helen Godfrey

FORM AND FUNCTION

❛There are underlying biological systems to which we respond on levels that are often unconscious or subconscious. The reason we enjoy things in nature is that we see an economy of means, simplicity, elegance and an essential rightness there. But all these natural templates, rich in pattern, order and beauty, are not the result of decision making by mankind and therefore lie beyond our definition. We may call them 'design', as if we were speaking of a tool or artifact created by humans. But this is to falsify the issue since the beauty we see in nature is something we ascribe to processes we often don't understand.❜

(Papanek 1984)

The human body is unusual in that the very thing we are trying to understand is what we are. The inside of our bodies seems mysterious, made up of weird and wonderful structures that are initially difficult to comprehend. On closer examination, however, it becomes apparent that the structure of each organ is intimately connected to its functions. A consideration of the structural attributes necessary to fulfil these functions effectively helps to explain why organs have their particular structure. That form relates to function is a key concept in biological sciences and leads to understanding complex structures rather than just describing them.

Form and function of organs and tissues

The relationship between form and function is illustrated at all levels of organization within our bodies. The human body is made up of a number of organ systems that all work in an integrated way to maintain health. The hierarchy of organizational levels within the human body can be illustrated by examining the components within the digestive system. The digestive system is a collection of organs, including the stomach, liver and small intestine, which are responsible for breaking down food and providing the necessary chemicals for individual cells to use. Each of these organs is a functional unit made up of a number of different tissues.

There are many different kinds of tissues in the human body, but each could be put into one of four main categories based on structure and function. These tissues (see Fig. 1.1) are the building blocks of the body, analogous to the building materials of a house, which in the right proportions and combinations construct the human body. Each organ is built from tissues most appropriate for its purpose. For example, the stomach is a muscular organ responsible for digesting food. All four main types of tissue, epithelial, connective, muscle and nervous tissue, are found in the stomach. Each tissue contributes in an integrated way to the functions of the stomach. In addition to the muscle tissue in the stomach wall, the lining is epithelial tissue specially adapted for secreting digestive juices. A network of nerve fibres is responsible for coordinating the activity of the muscle fibres, creating churning movements in the stomach. The outer layer of the stomach is connective tissue, which offers protection. The precise combination, organization and structure of these tissues in the stomach effectively illustrate the link between form and function (see Fig. 1.2).

Historically, knowledge of the inside of the human body began with the recognition that the body was constructed out of variously shaped balls, bags and tubes. These 'organs' were described as being surrounded by tissues and fibres making up the texture or 'matter' of the human body. It is now recognized that the basic unit of living matter is a cell and that tissues are collections of structurally and functionally similar cells.

Form and function of cells

Cells come in a huge variety of shapes and sizes and their forms reflect different functions. Smooth muscle cells found in the walls of hollow organs like the stomach are spindle-shaped reflecting their function, which is to shorten during contraction and lengthen during

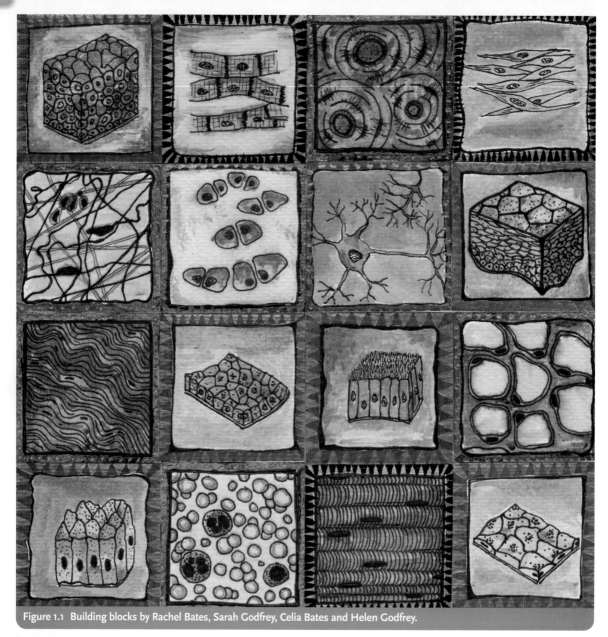

Figure 1.1 Building blocks by Rachel Bates, Sarah Godfrey, Celia Bates and Helen Godfrey.

Key to picture:

1	2	3	4
5	6	7	8
9	10	11	12
13	14	15	16

Epithelial tissues: 1: transitional epithelium, 8: stratified squamous epithelium, 10: cuboidal epithelium, 11: ciliated epithelium, 13: columnar epithelium and 16: squamous epithelium. Connective tissues: 3: compact bone, 5: areolar (loose connective) tissue, 6: hyaline cartilage, 9: fibrous connective tissue, 12: adipose tissue and 14: blood. Muscle tissues: 2: cardiac muscle, 4: smooth muscle and 15: skeletal muscle. Nervous tissue: 7: nervous tissue.

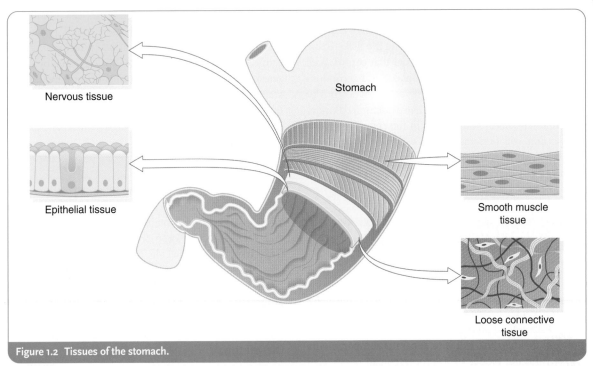

Figure 1.2 Tissues of the stomach.

A portion of the anterior wall has been cut away to reveal the different tissues found in the stomach wall. These include the four major tissue types: epithelial, connective, muscle and nervous tissues.

relaxation. They are called 'smooth' muscle cells because they lack the stripes or striations found in muscle cells of the heart and skeletal muscle.

The design of a cell relates to its function and this concept of 'form and function' is also fundamental to the design of many objects. For example, the design of a chair is influenced by its potential function. Consider the design criteria for a stool to perch on for a few minutes with that of a seat to sink into and relax for a couple of hours. The stool does not have to be as comfortable as the seat. Obviously the analogy between chair design and 'cell form' has limitations; a designer also considers the aesthetic pleasure the chair will give (see Fig. 1.3).

Using this concept of form relating to function in understanding the structure of cells, it can be deduced that nerve cells are long and thin so that they can carry messages in the form of nerve impulses over relatively long distances. Red blood cells are small and biconcave in shape. The shape and other characteristics of red blood cells, such as their lack of a nucleus, can be attributed to their function of carrying oxygen around the body. Dispensing with a nucleus enables more haemoglobin, the oxygen-carrying pigment, to be crammed into a red blood cell so that more oxygen can be carried. The flattened shape of the red blood cell provides a large

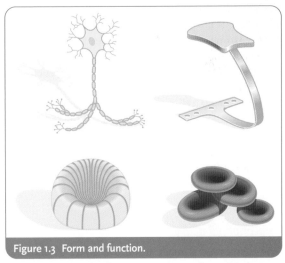

Figure 1.3 Form and function.

Nerve cells and red blood cells are structurally modified to perform their unique functions. The design of a chair also illustrates the concept of form and function.

surface area over which oxygen can enter by diffusion, a mechanism that will be explained later in this chapter.

Although there are many different cell 'forms' reflecting their particular functions, there are three main parts common to virtually all cells. The plasma membrane surrounds the cell and controls the entry and exit of material from its immediate watery environment, the tissue fluid. The nucleus contains genetic material that controls cell division and metabolism. The cytoplasm is a semi-fluid medium in which many of the cell's activities occur. The cytoplasm contains organelles, small structural components that have specific functions in the cell. The following section will demonstrate how the cell membrane and cell organelles illustrate the unity between form and function.

Form and function within cells

Cell membrane

The plasma, or cell membrane is the outer boundary that protects the fragile chemistry of the cytoplasm from its surroundings. Membranes are also present inside the cell, dividing the cell into separate compartments where different biochemical processes can occur. Cell membranes control the entry and exit of a variety of chemicals and are actively engaged in important chemical reactions.

Although the cell membrane is only about 12 nm in thickness (1 nm is 10^{-9} m or $1/1000\,000\,000$ m) it is very strong. The membrane surrounding the cell or an organelle is fatty in nature, which seems strange given that the body is a very watery environment and fats and water are not natural partners. However, the fatty part of the cell membrane is made up of special lipid molecules called phospholipids. A lipid is another name for fat; phospholipids are fatty molecules containing phosphate. Each phospholipid molecule has two parts, the phosphate 'head', which is 'water loving' or hydrophilic, and the 'tail', which is 'water hating' or hydrophobic.

Phospholipid bilayer

The membrane is made up of two layers of phospholipids, known as a bilayer, with the lipid parts in the middle. The hydrophobic 'tails' consisting of hydrocarbon chains are sandwiched in the middle by the hydrophilic 'heads' exposed on the two surfaces (see Fig. 1.4). This means that the fatty filling of this sandwich-like structure is not in contact with the watery environment. Fatty molecules can go through the membrane relatively easily whilst water soluble molecules have to go through special channels or pores.

A key feature of the model of the cell membrane suggested by Singer and Nicholson (1972) is that the phospholipid bilayer contains various proteins straddled across the phospholipid bilayer to a greater or lesser extent (see Fig. 1.4). Small amounts of carbohydrate are attached to some proteins and lipids within the membrane; these are called glycoproteins and glycolipids and are found on the outside of the cell's outer membrane, the plasma membrane.

Protein molecules

Protein molecules in the cell membrane perform a variety of functions, and include protein channels, protein 'pumps' and carrier proteins to transport substances in and out of the cell. Some proteins, called cell adhesion molecules, enable the cells to stick to each other. They are important to prevent cells wandering off during development and ending up in the wrong place. On the other hand, some cells do need to migrate; when cells inappropriately wander or stick together they may either cause or contribute to deterioration in certain diseases (Newell 1992).

Many proteins in the cell membrane act as receptors for signalling molecules, such as hormones, and others act as cell markers, which let other cells in the body know that they are 'self' rather than 'non-self'. This is an important attribute for an effective immune system, which needs to detect invading microorganisms. These cell markers are glycoproteins and together with glycolipids play an important role in establishing cellular identity.

The cell membrane, because of its composition and particular arrangement, controls materials that pass through it. If a cell was totally impermeable or totally permeable life would be impossible. The environment within the cell can only remain stable if a cell is able to take in raw materials from the surroundings and pass wastes and other chemicals out into the environment. It is important that only some substances are allowed to pass through, so the cell membrane is said to be selectively- or semi-permeable.

Transport of substances across the cell membrane

Materials can be transported across cell membranes in a variety of ways. The simplest are the movement of individual molecules across the cell membrane by diffusion and osmosis. Diffusion is the passive movement of molecules from a region of high concentration to a region where they are at a lower concentration. Osmosis is a special case of diffusion in which water flows across a selectively permeable membrane from a region where

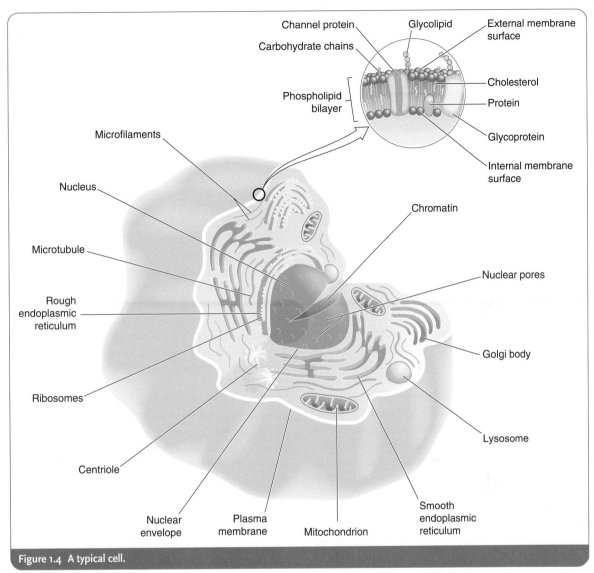

Figure 1.4 A typical cell.

An artist's interpretation of cell structure illustrating the variety of cell organelles and the structure of the plasma membrane. The plasma membrane is composed of a phospholipid bilayer studded with a variety of protein molecules.

water is at a high concentration to a region where water is at a lower concentration.

There are various channels and pumps in cell membranes that enable specific materials to enter or leave. Different cells will have particular kinds of channels and pumps, depending on their function, allowing only certain substances to enter or leave. Some proteins in the cell membrane may bind with and help or facilitate the diffusion of molecules across the cell membrane; this process is called carrier-mediated transport or facilitated diffusion. Sometimes energy is required to move particles across the cell membrane against a concentration gradient, this is called active transport. Proteins involved in active transport are often called 'pumps'.

Large suspended molecules can be taken into the cell by a mechanism called phagocytosis, which involves a relatively large solid mass such as a bacterium being engulfed by the cell, and being digested or broken down. This process of taking material in is also called endocytosis. Substances can be removed from the cell by the same mechanism in reverse, called exocytosis. Much smaller amounts of fluid containing dissolved or suspended substances can be brought into the cell by pinocytosis, which is similar to phagocytosis, but on a much smaller scale.

The fluid and dynamic structure of the cell membrane clearly relates to its functions; this relationship is also reflected by other components within the cell. The cell is the basic unit of living matter and it exhibits the same characteristics of multi-cellular organisms including nutrition, respiration, growth, excretion, responding to stimuli and reproduction. These cell activities are supported by various cell organelles whose form (see Fig. 1.4) also relates to function.

Cell organelles

The cytoplasm contains an abundance of weird and wonderfully shaped components, various granules, sacs and labyrinthine networks of membranes (see Fig. 1.5). These are described next.

Endoplasmic reticulum

Numerous and diverse activities are possible in cells due to the presence of membranes, which form boundaries dividing the cell into separate compartments. These membranes form a 'network' within the cell, which is what the word 'reticulum' literally means. The form of the endoplasmic reticulum relates to its function, which is to make and transport substances within the cell. Rough endoplasmic reticulum is covered with groups of ribosomes, tiny spherical structures responsible for synthesizing proteins. Smooth endoplasmic reticulum is smooth in appearance because it lacks ribosomes. The role of smooth endoplasmic reticulum varies in different cells, but it is always devoted to synthesizing non-protein substances. The rough endoplasmic reticulum synthesizes proteins, which can then be moved within the membrane to where they are required in the cell. Proteins contain structural information that signposts them to their correct location (Hopkins 1989). Optimum cell function relies on proteins being in the right place, if these proteins contain incorrect markers they may end up in the wrong place and be eventually destroyed. This problem occurs in certain inherited diseases, including cystic fibrosis (Olkkonen & Ikonen 2000). The genetic basis of cystic fibrosis is discussed in Chapter 10.

Golgi body

As manufactured molecules move from one compartment to another they can be modified. For example, proteins destined to move out of the rough endoplasmic reticulum move onto another cell organelle involved in processing materials, the Golgi body. As they pass through the Golgi body many proteins have sugars and amino acids tagged on (Hopkins 1989).

The Golgi body, named after Camillo Golgi, an Italian neuroscientist, is structurally and functionally related to the endoplasmic reticulum. The Golgi body is made up of a stack of about five flattened membranous sacs. This organelle is part of the cell's processing and transport machinery, and is responsible for sorting and delivering proteins, carbohydrates and lipids to the right places within the cell. Secretory products that are destined to leave the cell are pinched off into secretory vesicles and leave the cell by exocytosis.

Lysosomes

Lysosomes are literally bags of enzymes originating from the Golgi body. Enzymes are proteins that control chemical reactions taking place in the body (see p. 32). The lysosomal membrane is slightly thicker to protect the cell from its lethal enzymes. The various enzymes are responsible for breaking down larger molecules originating inside or outside the cell, to smaller component parts. The lysosome is a bit like the cell's waste disposal and recycling centre, its main role being to remove and degrade unwanted or damaged macromolecules such as proteins, carbohydrates, fats and nucleic acids (Lloyd 1990).

Macromolecules from outside the cell are brought into contact with lysosomes inside the cell by phagocytosis and pinocytosis. As suggested earlier, these two processes are similar in some respects, but phagocytosis only occurs in certain cells called phagocytes whereas most cells engage in pinocytosis.

Phagocytes contribute to immune defences in the lung tissues; scavenging phagocytes called macrophages ingest and degrade any bacteria inhaled in the air. Certain substances that cells bring inside through phagocytosis and pinocytosis cannot be broken down. These include small particles of silica inhaled during industrial exposure in occupations such as mining, quarrying and stone cutting. These particles accumulate in the phagocytes within the lung tissues, where they interact with the lysosomal membrane, which ultimately breaks down and releases enzymes into the cytoplasm causing the cell to be digested and die. Fibrous nodules form in the lungs, which gradually cause lung destruction and respiratory symptoms (Greaves 1994).

Dysfunction of lysosomes is also implicated in certain neurodegenerative disorders including Alzheimer's disease (see p. 62). In Alzheimer's disease the breakdown of membrane proteins by lysosomes is disturbed, leading to the accumulation of protein fragments within nerve cells. These aggregates called amyloid cause the lysosome to burst, releasing enzymes, which ultimately

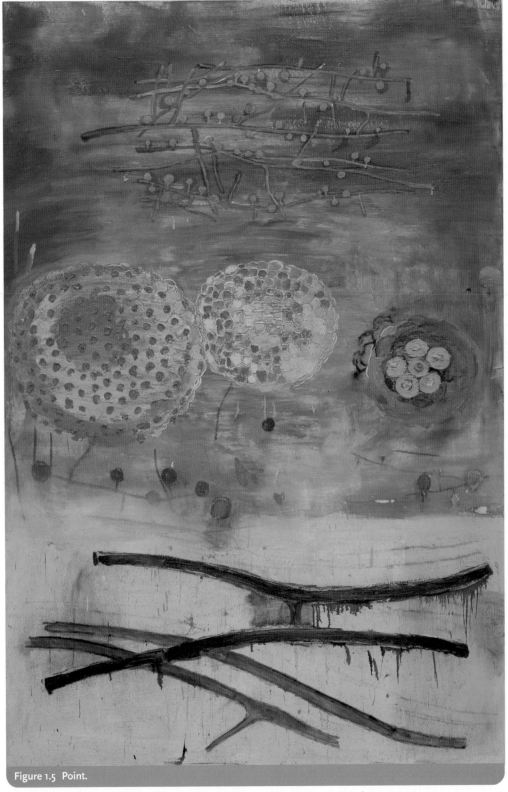

Figure 1.5 Point.

Terry Winters, 'oil on linen' painted in 1985. (Reproduced with kind permission of Terry Winters.)

destroy the nerve cells. This process leads to the formation of neuritic plaques found in the brains of individuals with Alzheimer's disease (Mayer 1993).

Microtubules and microfilaments

Weaving through the cytoplasm of cells is an elaborate network of hollow tubes and solid fibres often referred to as the cytoskeleton. The different shapes of cells, their mobility, and their ability to change shape and move components around inside the cell relies on a particular cell organelle called a microtubule. Microtubules are very small tubes that exist alone or in elaborately arranged groups. Bundles of microtubules are found in precise arrangements within cilia (short thin processes), flagella (long processes) and mitotic spindles formed from centrioles during cell division. Microtubules are dynamic structures constructed from proteins called tubulins which can be built up into longer microtubules or broken down into smaller microtubules (Gull 1990). Drugs used in the treatment of some cancers are based on their ability to bind to tubulin proteins. The tubulin proteins are disabled and unable to form microtubules. This disturbs the formation of the mitotic spindle, a framework that separates chromosomes in a precise way during cell division (see p. 113). These drugs therefore inhibit cell division (Gull 1990).

Microfilaments are smaller and composed of a protein called actin. Actin filaments are associated with myosin filaments in muscle cells in a highly organized way. They cause muscle contraction as they slide over each other (see Ch. 5).

Mitochondria

In all human cells that contain a nucleus there are cell organelles called mitochondria. Mitochondria have a double membrane like the nucleus and even possess their own DNA molecule. This suggests that mitochondria lived independently in the early history of life on earth. Mitochondria are the sites of energy production in cells. The energy is produced in the form of adenosine triphosphate (ATP) which is the 'energy currency' necessary to drive cell activities. The number of mitochondria in a cell usually depends on the cell's energy requirements. Cells that use a lot of energy, such as muscle cells, may have thousands of mitochondria.

Mitochondria are often sausage shaped, usually about 0.2 μm in diameter and 5 μm in length. The structure of a mitochondrion is well suited to its function. The energy produced in mitochondria results from the breakdown of food molecules by enzymes. The enzymes that drive this controlled release of energy are located on the inner mitochondrial membrane. The inner membrane has an expansive surface area to accommodate large numbers of enzymes and therefore folds to fit into the outer membrane.

Mitochondrial DNA codes for some of the proteins found in the inner mitochondrial membrane. These proteins form part of the enzyme complexes involved in the production of energy. Mitochondrial DNA mutates (changes in structure) more quickly than the DNA in the cell nucleus probably due to the production of oxygen radicals, which are highly reactive particles that can damage mitochondrial DNA (Kirkwood 2002). Changes in the mitochondrial DNA are thought to be a significant feature of the ageing process (see p. 117) (Walker 1994). Problems with producing energy may be an important feature of neurodegenerative diseases such as Alzheimer's and Parkinson's diseases. Falling levels of ATP production activates enzymes that alter a protein called tau protein inside brain cells, ultimately leading to neurofibrillary tangles. The formation of neurofibrillary tangles within brain cells involves microtubules introduced earlier in this chapter. The microtubules become altered in structure and function in these neurofibrillary tangles leading to brain cell dysfunction (Walker 1994, St. George-Hyslop 2000).

Thus, mutations in the mitochondrial DNA acquired during life are implicated in ageing and neurodegenerative diseases (Wallace 1999). In addition there are many other diseases that are linked to mutations of mitochondrial DNA. Some of these mutations are sporadic and others are transmitted down the maternal line (Chinnery & Turnbull 1999).

Nucleus

The nucleus is responsible for coordinating and controlling cell activities so that cell homeostasis, or harmony, is maintained. The nucleus stores genetic information in the DNA molecules, which become tightly coiled within chromosomes during cell division (see Ch. 10). This includes instructions to make specific enzymes that control chemical reactions in the cell to ensure homeostasis and health are maintained. The structure of the nucleus is well suited to these two functions. In cells that are not dividing, the genetic material, which is a thread-like mass of DNA called chromatin, is protected by a double nuclear membrane. Communication between the cytoplasm and the nucleoplasm, the jelly-like substance found in the nucleus, is possible via nuclear pores. The outer layer of the nuclear membrane is continuous with the endoplasmic reticulum and plasma membrane

Table 1.1 Organelles and their functions	
Organelle	*Function*
Nucleus	Stores DNA, controls cellular activities
Ribosomes	Sites of protein synthesis
Rough endoplasmic reticulum	Contributes to synthesis and transport of proteins
Smooth endoplasmic reticulum	Synthesis of non-protein substances such as lipids
Golgi body	Processing and packaging of lipids and proteins
Lysosomes	Digestion of harmful substances and waste material
Microtubules and microfilaments	Forms the cytoskeleton which provides structural support and allows movement
Mitochondria	Production of energy (ATP) for the cell

so that the nucleus may communicate with the tissue fluid.

In summary, the key cell functions include energy production, synthesis of new materials, processing and transport of materials, recycling and waste disposal, movement and coordination of activities. These activities are performed by various cell organelles working in an integrated way (see Table 1.1). Each organelle's form relates to its function. In the next section various aspects of the structure and function of cells, tissues and organs in the digestive system are explored to emphasize the relationship between form and function on a somewhat larger scale.

Introducing the digestive system

Humans, like other animals, get their energy from food. The digestive system is responsible for breaking down food so that its stored energy can be used by all the cells in the body. The digestive system is literally a long tube about 10 m in length, stretching from the mouth to the anus with some associated glands, whose secretions are passed to the lumen of the tract via ducts. These additional glands are the salivary glands, the liver and gall bladder, and the pancreas (see Fig. 1.6).

The structure or form of the gut is well suited to its functions. The basic structure of the digestive tract is adapted in different anatomical regions to perform the physiological functions of ingestion, digestion, absorption, assimilation and defecation. For example, the tube becomes dilated in the stomach so that food can be stored between meals, while the small intestine is very long, providing a large surface area for absorption of the products of digestion.

The long tube, or gastrointestinal tract, is punctuated by various sphincters (rings of smooth muscle) and valves. This ensures that food is propelled in a controlled way in one direction only.

Four-layer structure of gut wall

Despite being differentiated along its length, the gut wall has the same four main layers throughout; these are the mucosa, submucosa, muscle layer and serosa, and each has a particular form and function.

Mucosa

The mucosa is the innermost layer and is in contact with the food as it passes through the lumen of the tract. It is highly folded to increase the surface area available for digestion and absorption. The mucosa is made up of epithelium, loose connective tissue and a thin layer of smooth muscle. The lining epithelium is in contact with the gut contents; it is thicker in areas prone to friction, such as the mouth, oesophagus and rectum, and consists of many layers of epithelial cells, stratified squamous epithelium. Where the gut contents are more fluid and there is less risk of abrasion, the epithelium is thinner and is made up of a single layer of columnar (column-shaped) epithelial cells. Mucus is secreted by goblet cells, and this lubricates and protects the mucosa.

Submucosa

A thin layer of smooth muscle separates the mucosa from the submucosa and is responsible for movements of the folds of mucosa in the lumen. The submucosa consists of loose connective tissue and is rich in blood vessels and lymph vessels. It contains part of a plexus, or network of autonomic nerve fibres, involved in the control of gastrointestinal secretions.

Muscle layer

The muscle layer consists of two thick sheets of smooth muscle, an inner sheet of circular fibres and an outer sheet of longitudinal fibres. The two layers contract antagonistically and cause peristalsis – slow wave-like

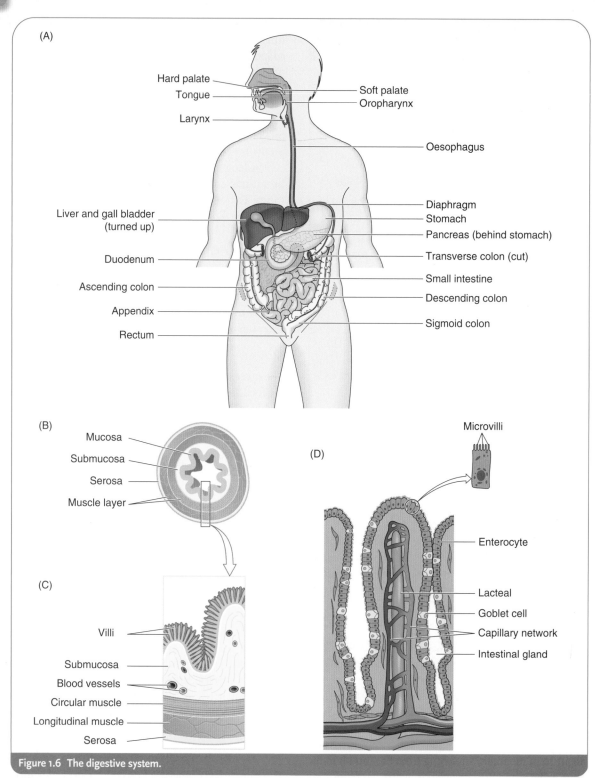

Figure 1.6 The digestive system.

(A) This shows the structures of the digestive tract and associated glands. (B) The structure of the gut wall is made up of four layers. (C) In the small intestine the folds of mucosa are covered with villi. (D) Each villus is covered with epithelial cells which possess microvilli. This 'brush border' increases the surface area for absorption of digested food products. (Parts (A) and (D) reproduced with kind permission from Waugh & Grant 2001.)

contractions that mix and propel the gut contents along. A large network of autonomic nerve fibres on the outer surface of the muscle layer control motility (movement) of the gut.

Serosa

The serosa is the outermost layer of the gut wall and consists of squamous epithelium and loose connective tissue. It forms part of the peritoneum, a double-layered membrane that drapes over abdominal organs and lines the whole of the abdominal cavity.

The four major types of tissue – epithelial, connective, muscle and nervous tissue – introduced earlier in the chapter are all found in precise combinations within the four layers of the gut wall, once again illustrating how form relates to function (see Fig. 1.6).

Activities in the gut

The conversion of food into a form suitable for use by cells involves the gut performing a number of key processes. Food has to be first eaten, or ingested, and then digested, or broken down into smaller molecules. Chemical digestion is accomplished by digestive enzymes and mechanical digestion by chewing, churning and pulverizing food into smaller particles. The small, soluble molecules resulting from digestion are absorbed from the digestive tract, mainly through the small intestine, into the blood and lymph vessels. Blood containing these products of digestion is then transported to the liver. These molecules are assimilated into the body for use or storage by cells. Indigestible substances in food such as fibre, the cellulose from plant cell walls, are eliminated from the body in faeces. The main organs of the gastrointestinal tract that perform these functions will be introduced next to illustrate key features of their form and functions.

Form and function of the stomach

The stomach is adapted to perform many important functions. It receives food from the oesophagus, mixes it with gastric juice, begins the process of digesting proteins, absorbs small quantities of water, electrolytes, glucose, alcohol and certain drugs, and passes food onto the small intestine.

The stomach is a pouch-like organ that can hold large volumes of swallowed food for a few hours. Once food enters the stomach, gentle peristaltic movements mix it with gastric juice producing a liquid called chyme.

The stomach churns the food in a particular way because the muscle layer has an additional layer of oblique muscle fibres. The three-dimensional muscle movements enhance digestion. Both the churning and secretion of gastric juice are controlled by the vagus nerve. An increase in nerve impulses along parasympathetic fibres (see Ch. 6) within the vagus nerve stimulate both chemical secretion and muscle movements (Hoyle 1997).

Gastric juice is produced by glands in the gastric pits that stud the inner lining mucosa of the stomach. Each gland possesses different types of specialized secretory cells. For example, oxyntic (parietal) cells secrete hydrochloric acid that destroys bacteria present in the ingested food and activates precursor enzymes secreted by chief (zymogen) cells. Goblet cells secrete mucus that coats the mucosa and protects it from acid and protein-digesting enzymes. Intrinsic factor is also secreted by specialized cells and is needed for vitamin B_{12} absorption. Vitamin B_{12} is necessary for red blood cell production, and the absence of this factor causes pernicious anaemia (Hoyle 1997).

Form and function in the small intestine

The small intestine is a very long tubular organ consisting of three parts, the duodenum, jejunum and ileum. The small intestine is well adapted to its functions of digestion and absorption. Chyme is passed from the stomach to the duodenum a little at a time through the relaxation of the smooth muscle of the pyloric sphincter. A sphincter is a circular muscle that closes an opening or, as in this case, the lumen of a tubular structure. The short C-shaped duodenum receives bile and pancreatic juice via another sphincter, the sphincter of Oddi.

Digestion in the small intestine

Bile is a fluid produced by liver cells and stored in the gall bladder. Bile contains bile salts that transform large volumes of fat into many tiny microscopic particles with an increased surface area. This process, called emulsification, enhances the actions of lipases, enzymes that digest lipids. Alkaline pancreatic juice facilitates the actions of the digestive enzymes in the small intestine and helps neutralize the acidic chyme.

Digestion of food is completed in the small intestine by enzymes embedded in the surfaces of microvilli present in the columnar epithelial cells. These enzymes finish the digestion of food molecules just prior to absorption. The end products of protein digestion are amino acids. Carbohydrate-digesting enzymes release monosaccharides from carbohydrates, lipases split lipids into glycerol and fatty acids, and nucleases break down nucleic acids.

It is important that the secretions of enzymes into the lumen of the gut occur in a coordinated way, as it would be wasteful if enzymes were released in the absence of food. In addition, the timing of gut movements needs to be coordinated so that the gut contents are shunted along at the appropriate speed for optimum digestion and absorption. Gut activity is coordinated by parasympathetic branches of the vagus nerve and various hormones. Whenever the synchrony of events is disrupted, pain and discomfort are experienced (Burdett 1991).

Usually, thick mucus protects the mucosal lining against autodigestion by digestive juices. Pain in the gut can also result from peptic ulcers, which are areas in the mucosa exposed to acid and protein-digesting enzymes. Peptic ulcers commonly occur in the stomach and duodenum, where the gut contents are most acid. One of the most common factors associated with peptic ulcer formation is the presence of *Helicobacter pylori* infection. The bacteria selectively bind to the surface of mucus-secreting epithelial cells in the stomach and are able to withstand the acidic environment by secreting an enzyme that makes their immediate environment more alkaline. The bacteria are resilient to the host immune responses and are difficult to eradicate completely with antimicrobial therapy (Podolski 1996).

Absorption

The small intestine is perfectly designed to absorb the end products of digestion. Intestinal fluid provides a medium for the digestive products facilitating absorption across the intestinal mucosa. The surface area of the small intestine is very large because of its long length and because the intestinal lining is thrown into circular folds. The mucosa also has numerous villi, finger-like projections that with the epithelial 'brush border', or microvilli, increase the surface area and facilitate absorption (see Fig. 1.6). Each villus has an extensive blood and lymphatic supply; most molecules are absorbed into the blood whilst some products of digestion, the long-chain fatty acids, are absorbed into the lymphatic circulation. Absorption of materials occurs through the epithelial membranes of villi via a number of mechanisms including diffusion, osmosis, active transport and pinocytosis. Thus, the small intestine is beautifully adapted to absorb

water, electrolytes and the molecules of digestion. It has a large surface area and a very adequate means of transporting absorbed molecules away from the gut.

Form and function of the large intestine

The large intestine is approximately 1.5 m in length; it is called 'large' because of its greater diameter. The large intestine appears as a series of pouches resulting from the precise arrangement of the longitudinal muscle into three bands rather than a sheet of muscle as elsewhere in the gut. These muscle bands act a bit like pieces of elastic gathering up material at the waist of a skirt. The large intestine has four main areas, the caecum, colon, rectum and anal canal.

There are several functions of the large intestine that contribute to homeostasis and health. These include storage of undigested matter until it is eliminated. Absorption in the large intestine is mainly limited to water, electrolytes (principally sodium) and vitamins. Ninety per cent of the water that enters the large intestine is absorbed. Consolidation of faeces occurs as water is absorbed in the caecum and colon. Faeces are eliminated by a mechanism called defecation.

Role of bacteria

The large intestine also contains a resident bacterial population that contribute to health. Certain bacteria synthesize vitamins including vitamin K, B_{12}, thiamine and riboflavine. Bacteria such as Lactobacilli and Bifidobacteria are thought to stimulate the gut immune response, lower cholesterol and triglycerides in the blood, and also lessen the risk of cancer. These bacteria are encouraged to flourish in the gut when yoghurts containing live bacteria are eaten. Certain types of carbohydrate, oligosaccharides found in peas, beans, garlic, onions and cereals are also thought to enhance their growth (Cummings 1995).

Starches resistant to digestion are found in beans, peas, lentils, pasta and whole grain cereals. This resistant starch is beneficial to health because it takes longer to digest and provokes much lower blood glucose and insulin responses after a meal. These resistant starches are digested in the first part of the large intestine, the caecum, rather than the small intestine by the resident bacteria. Other dietary carbohydrates, the oligosaccharides and dietary fibre are also digested in the large intestine. Bacteria in the caecum break down these carbohydrates to a variety of compounds including butyrate, which is thought to protect against cancer of the large intestine. The bacteria add biomass to the faeces and increase faecal bulk thereby influencing bowel habits and preventing constipation (Cummings 1995).

A further bonus is that when these 'good' bacteria thrive they may inhibit the growth of potentially harmful bacteria in the gut. Gut bacteria are not just passive occupants, they are thought to communicate with gut cells so that an intimate relationship between bacteria and gut cells is established (Hamilton 1999).

It is apparent that the digestive system carries out a complex series of physiological mechanisms made possible by a range of anatomical structures; cells, tissues and organs exquisitely adapted to perform specific tasks.

References

Burdett K 1991 A question of timing: effective digestion. Biological Sciences Review 3(4):37–41

Chinnery P F, Turnbull D M 1999 Mitochondrial DNA and disease. Lancet 354(1S) Supplement:17S1–21S1

Cummings J 1995 A new look at dietary carbohydrates. MRC News 68:36–40

Greaves I A 1994 Occupational pulmonary diseases. In: McCunney R J (ed). A practical approach to occupational and environmental medicine, 2nd edn. Little, Brown & Co., Boston, p 145–165

Gull K 1990 Microtubules. The cell's most dynamic organelles? Biological Sciences Review 2(5):8–22

Hamilton G 1999 Insider training. New Scientist 162(2192): 42–46

Hopkins C 1989 Passports and passengers protein traffic in cells. Biological Sciences Review 1(4):18–22

Hoyle T 1997 The digestive system: linking theory and practice. British Journal of Nursing 6(22):1285–1291

Kirkwood T 2002 Unravelling the mysteries of ageing. Biological Sciences Review 14(3):33–37

Lloyd J 1990 Lysosomes. Biological Sciences Review 3(2):21–24

Mayer J 1993 Brain disease and ageing. Biological Sciences Review 5(3):28–30

Newell J 1992 A sticky end for disease. New Scientist 136(1850):29–31

Olkkonen V M, Ikonen E 2000 Mechanisms of disease: genetic defects of intracellular-membrane transport. New England Journal of Medicine 343(15):1095–1104

Papanek V 1984 Design for the real world. 2nd edn. Thames & Hudson, London, p 4

Podolski J L 1996 Recent advances in peptic ulcer disease: Helicobacter pylori infection and its treatment. Gastroenterological Nursing 19(4):128–136

St. George-Hyslop P H 2000 Piecing together Alzheimer's. Scientific American 283(6):52–59

Singer S J, Nicholson G L 1972 The fluid mosaic model: the structure of cell membrane. Science 175:720–732

Wallace D C 1999 Mitochondrial diseases in mouse and man. Science 283:1482–1488

Walker J 1994 The power behind the cell. MRC News 64:10–13

Waugh A, Grant A 2001 Ross and Wilson: Anatomy and physiology in health and illness. Churchill Livingstone, Edinburgh

2

HOMEOSTASIS

> ❝ In traditional medicine, ... health is a state of precarious balance – being threatened, toppled and restored – between the body, the universe and society. More important than curing is the aim of preventing imbalance from occurring in the first place. Equilibrium is to be achieved by avoiding excess and pursuing moderation. ❞

(Porter 1997)

In this quotation, 'traditional medicine' refers to medicine based on popular beliefs about the body, health and disease rather than Western scientific medicine.

Homeostasis is a key concept in physiology that explains how and why the body is able to adapt to change. It is a state of balance and stability within the body irrespective of environmental changes. Many factors affect the suitability of body fluids within the internal environment to sustain life, including temperature, acidity, salinity and the concentration of nutrients and wastes. These properties affect the chemical reactions carried out by cells that keep us alive and so there are physiological mechanisms to keep them at appropriate levels. Homeostasis describes all the processes that provide the maintenance of conditions under which cells and therefore the body can function properly.

Claude Bernard, a French physiologist, began to develop this concept of homeostasis in the middle of the nineteenth century. Bernard was hugely influential in experimental medicine and his work covered many aspects including experimental work (see Fig. 2.1) which led to the understanding that physiology was the scientific basis for medicine (Porter 1997). Bernard recognized the importance of the constancy of the internal environment for free life (Buchman 1996, Rinomhota & Cooper 1996). Walter Cannon, an

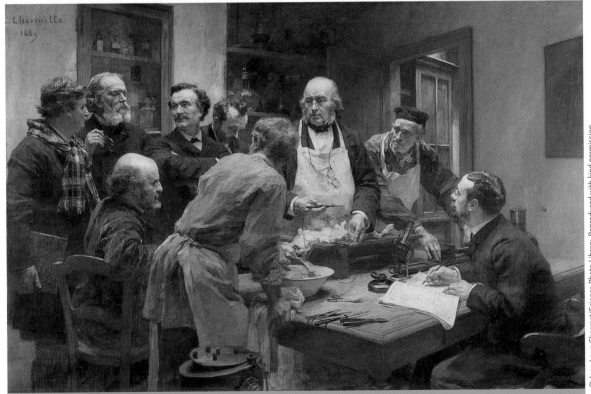

Figure 2.1 Claude Bernard in his laboratory.

American physiologist, introduced the term 'homeostasis', which literally means 'staying the same'. Cannon understood that the body's internal environment did not literally 'stay the same', and recognized that homeostasis is about maintaining a relatively constant environment. Homeostasis provides a basis for health, since these relatively constant conditions ensure optimum cell and tissue function. Illness occurs due to change in some aspect of the internal environment (McVicar & Clancy 1998).

Tissues are made up of collections of cells bathed in tissue fluid, a watery medium derived from blood. Tissue fluid is an extracellular fluid (i.e. found outside cells) that constitutes the internal environment. Cells will only function efficiently if this tissue fluid is kept relatively constant. Since cell function demands the use of a constant supply of materials and leads to the production of metabolic waste products, components within the tissue fluid are continually changing. The stability of this liquid environment depends on a dynamic equilibrium or balance between inputs and outputs.

The cell activities outlined in Chapter 1 depend on cells having access to a continual supply of raw materials and being able to get rid of metabolic waste. All cells require energy in the form of ATP to drive activities; energy is produced in mitochondria as a result of cell respiration. This process requires oxygen and glucose, so the levels of these two variables must remain relatively constant for cells to function effectively. Transport of materials into and out of cells across cell membranes is affected by the osmotic pressure of the tissue fluid. Osmotic pressure is the amount of pressure needed to stop osmosis and therefore needs to be kept within a homeostatic range.

Enzymes control all biological processes and work best at a certain temperature and pH. Therefore the core body temperature and pH of tissue fluid need to be regulated so that cells can operate efficiently and survival can be assured. These and other factors are called physiological variables, they include the volume, temperature and various chemical constituents of tissue fluid; all have an effect on cell function and must be controlled by homeostatic mechanisms. Homeostasis is the goal of all the body's physiological processes. Being healthy depends on our ability to maintain a relatively constant internal environment so that cells, tissues, organs and organ systems can function optimally.

The concept of health reflecting a 'balance' or equilibrium in the body and illness reflecting disharmony has some resonance with traditional Chinese and Indian medicine and historically with the Greek concepts of humours. The Greeks believed illness occurred when one of the humours, blood, phlegm, black bile or yellow bile, dominated. In Chinese medicine the balance between *yin* and *yang* are central, whilst in traditional Indian medicine it is the balance between the opposing forces of *kapha* and *pitt*, mediated by *vata*, that is crucial (Kaptchuk & Croucher 1986).

Homeostatic systems

It is important to recognize that homeostasis is not just about maintaining relative constancy, but about responding to change (McVicar & Clancy 1998). Homeostatic systems have in-built control mechanisms that respond to change by producing responses that will themselves also lead to change. An important principle of homeostasis is that it is dynamic with self-adjusting mechanisms operating continuously. A homeostatic system has three linked components through which information flows continuously. This is often described as a feedback loop (see Fig. 2.2). In this the receptors detect changes in the variable and feed information to the controller, which integrates the information and compares it to the usual pre-programmed level, the set point value. The controller then feeds information to the effectors, which perform actions returning the variable towards the set point value.

Regulation of the internal environment is achieved by hormonal and neural mechanisms which coordinate the activities of all organ systems. The receptors are often, but not exclusively, nervous receptors and the

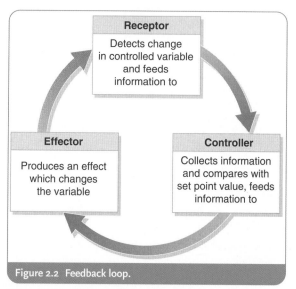

Figure 2.2 Feedback loop.

There are three components in every feedback control loop: a receptor, a controller and an effector.

controllers may be nervous or hormonal. The effectors in homeostatic mechanisms are various cells, tissues and organs that carry out the responses. This illustrates that all parts of the body are involved in homeostasis and that integrated functioning of all organ systems and physiological systems is necessary in the maintenance of homeostasis and health (Rinomhota & Cooper 1996).

A key concept in homeostasis is negative feedback in which fluctuations in the variable under control lead to changes occurring in the opposite direction. The principles of negative feedback are illustrated in glucose homeostasis. Blood glucose levels are controlled so that an increase in blood glucose, operating through receptors, controllers and effectors, causes responses that decrease blood glucose levels. So, if there is too much glucose, more of the hormone insulin will be secreted from the islets of Langerhans in the pancreas and the blood glucose levels will fall. Alternatively, if there is too little glucose, less insulin will be secreted and the amount of blood glucose in blood will rise (see Fig. 2.3). In other words, changes in blood glucose levels are reversed or negated, demonstrating the importance of negative feedback in resisting change and maintaining glucose, the variable, within a homeostatic range. This describes the principles of glucose homeostasis. In reality the mechanisms controlling blood glucose are more complex and involve a number of other hormones and several metabolic pathways.

Most homeostatic systems of the body are regulated by negative feedback mechanisms. Deviations from the norm or set point are resisted or negated. This tends to keep things relatively constant and allows homeostasis to be maintained. A slight deviation from the set point value will provoke negative feedback responses or corrective mechanisms that will tend to return the value back to the centre of the homeostatic range for that variable (Rinomhota & Cooper 1996).

There are some instances where a change from the norm is promoted rather than resisted. This is described as positive feedback and is usually a short-lived rapid response. Blood clotting is an example of a positive feedback mechanism that contributes to homeostasis by minimizing blood loss and ultimately maintaining the volume of tissue fluid. Blood clotting is initiated by a variety of factors and is a complex mechanism involving many clotting factors, although it can be summarized into three steps (see Fig. 2.4). The factors that initiate blood clotting appear in the blood in direct proportions to the extent of the tissue damage and once a blood clot forms it promotes more clotting; this self-initiating cascade action is an example of positive feedback (Wallis

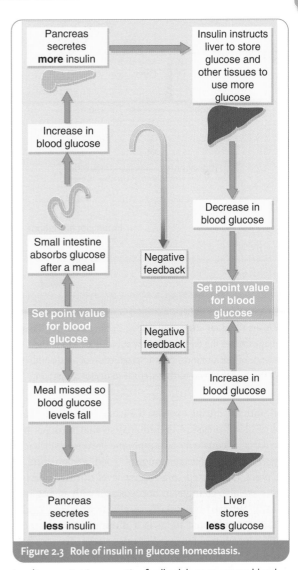

Figure 2.3 Role of insulin in glucose homeostasis.

Insulin operates in a negative feedback loop to ensure blood glucose levels remain fairly constant.

1994). Calcium ions are critical in this positive feedback mechanism; the amount of calcium ions appearing at the site of the blood clot is directly proportional to the tissue damage. The more calcium ions there are the greater the clot formation is, ensuring that the clot formed is appropriate to the extent of the tissue damage (see Fig. 2.5).

Therefore there are some positive feedback mechanisms, such as blood clotting, that do contribute to homeostasis. However, since homeostasis is about resisting change, most physiological systems incorporate negative feedback mechanisms as a means of maintaining stability (Rinomhota & Cooper 1996).

Another principle of homeostasis is that in certain circumstances it is necessary to modify the set point.

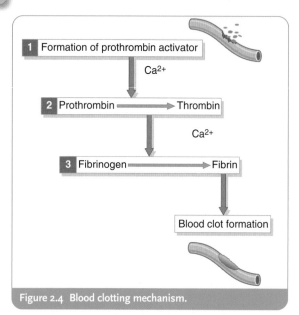

Figure 2.4 Blood clotting mechanism.

There are three key steps in the blood clotting cascade. Tissue damage causes the release of many substances and in the presence of calcium ions leads to production of prothrombin activator and then two further steps lead to clot formation.

For example, during exercise the usual homeostatic control of blood pressure is inhibited so that muscles will receive an adequate blood supply and therefore sufficient oxygen. The homeostatic range of blood pressure and its set point is adjusted to a higher level during exercise. There are also changes in homeostasis with ageing (see p. 118). Whilst homeostasis is still maintained under ambient conditions, there is a diminution in homeostatic control in older people under stress. This is characterized by a variable, such as osmotic pressure, moving further away from the set point and taking longer to return back to equilibrium than in younger people. This means, for example, that an older person may be more likely to become dehydrated due to difficulty in maintaining fluid balance (Dunbar 1996).

Regulation of body temperature

The regulation of body temperature is one of many homeostatic mechanisms that contribute to maintaining a state of inner balance. The control of body temperature is a good illustration of homeostasis and negative feedback mechanisms. A variety of cells, tissues and organs contribute to achieving a relatively constant core body temperature despite changes in the external environment.

Humans may encounter temperatures ranging from −50°C in Siberia to +50°C in African deserts. Whilst most of us are not exposed to such extremes of temperature we are able to tolerate significant temperature changes in our external environment and still maintain a core or deep body temperature within a homeostatic range of 36–38°C. The extremities, such as hands and feet, can get a lot colder than this without any adverse effects on homeostasis and health (Garland 1992). All the vital organs are found deep in the body; it is their temperature, and hence the core temperature, that needs to be kept within a narrow range close to 37°C.

Keeping the core body temperature fluctuating around 37°C is essential to ensure optimum cell function. Cell function depends on enzymes, and enzyme activity is inhibited at low temperatures. This is why we can delay food deterioration due to enzymes by chilling it in a fridge or can preserve it for longer by freezing. When enzymes are exposed to high temperatures, their structure changes and they can no longer function, so vital cell reactions cease. Structural change of enzymes and other proteins due to high temperatures is called denaturation. As an illustration of this, consider the changes that occur when an egg is cooked. The globular proteins become solid, an irreversible structural change. When enzyme-controlled reactions in cells fail as a result of temperature changes beyond the homeostatic range, the cells can no longer engage in crucial activities and ultimately die. Extreme temperature deviations lead to a failure of homeostasis and, eventually, death (Watson 1998).

A relatively constant core body temperature can only be achieved if the heat produced by the body or gained from the environment balances the heat lost. Heat is produced in chemical reactions occurring in cells. Most of this heat energy comes from the biochemical processes occurring in mitochondria, which convert food energy into ATP. Metabolic reactions that take place in the liver are a primary source of heat for the body. Skeletal muscle contractions also generate heat and shivering in adult humans is a key means of enhancing heat production. With adaptation to the cold, shivering disappears and other mechanisms are employed, including thermogenesis (production of heat) in brown adipose tissue (Lowell & Spiegelman 2000). Brown adipose tissue is a highly specialized fatty tissue with numerous mitochondria capable of producing large amounts of ATP (Rothwell 1989).

Blood transports heat around the body. The distribution of heat from the core to the periphery is crucial to the homeostatic mechanisms which regulate temperature in the body. The circulatory system determines the temperature of various parts of the body and the rate at which heat is lost via a number of mechanisms including radiation, evaporation, convection and conduction. Behavioural mechanisms such as adding or removing

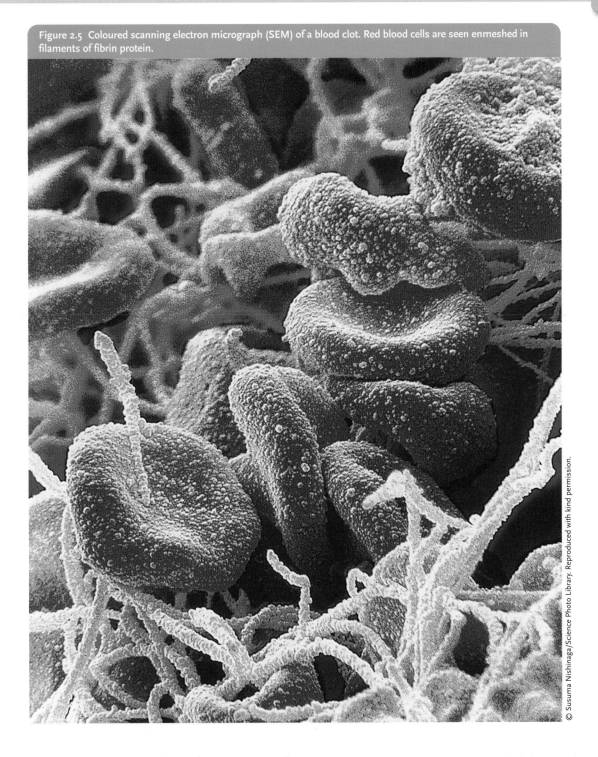

Figure 2.5 Coloured scanning electron micrograph (SEM) of a blood clot. Red blood cells are seen enmeshed in filaments of fibrin protein.

© Susuma Nishinaga/Science Photo Library. Reproduced with kind permission.

warm clothing enable us to enhance these processes of heat conservation and heat loss.

Heat transfer mechanisms

The skin plays an important role in temperature regulation because it is in touch with the external environment and provides a large surface area over which heat can be transferred to and from the environment. The most significant loss of heat from the body occurs via radiation and this depends on the difference in temperature between the skin and air: the steeper the temperature gradient the faster the heat loss. Conduction is the direct transfer of heat energy between two objects. For example, if someone sat on a cold concrete bench, they would lose heat. This route of heat loss can be important in the elderly following a fall and loss of consciousness.

Heat loss can occur by convection when wind moves the warm air away from the body. When it is windy the warm air surrounding the skin is continually replaced by cold air and this cools the body. Heat loss due to wind chill can be significant and the wind chill factor acknowledges the fact that heat loss is influenced by a combination of air temperature and wind velocity. Evaporation of sweat from the skin is another important route of heat loss. Heat energy is lost as water is converted to water vapour; this phenomenon is called cooling by evaporation.

Heat loss is an important consideration during surgery since it is estimated that up to 70% of patients undergoing surgery may lose heat and suffer an inadvertent drop in core temperature (Blackburn 1994). There are several factors that could contribute to heat loss including flimsy theatre gowns, draughty corridors, exposure of large parts of the body in theatre, administration of intravenous fluids cooler than body temperature and an inability to shiver while anaesthetized (Enright & Plowes 1999).

The temperature control systems use the same basic principle as all homeostatic systems: a controller receives information from receptors and activates mechanisms to resist the change (Rothwell 2000).

Thermoreceptors

Receptors that are sensitive to temperature change are called thermoreceptors. There are two types: heat receptors respond to temperatures above the core body temperature and cold receptors detect temperatures below that of the core temperature. Thermoreceptors are located in the periphery and in central areas within vital organs including the brain. Those in the skin are sensitive to temperature changes in the external environment and may be influential in eliciting behavioural responses to temperature change via the hypothalamus. Changes in the core temperature are monitored by thermoreceptors located in major organs and within an area of the hypothalamus called the preoptic area.

Temperature-regulating centre

The thermoreceptors send electrical signals to the hypothalamus, a small structure in the brain which plays a key role in homeostasis. The hypothalamus is at the centre of an integrated neural network involved in thermoregulation with links to the limbic system, brainstem, reticular formation, spinal cord and the sympathetic division of the autonomic nervous system (Mackowiak & Boulant 1996).

The hypothalamus compares the 'recorded' temperature to the set or preferred temperature and integrates this information with that received from thermoreceptors throughout the body. When the body temperature falls below the set point, the hypothalamus initiates activities to produce heat and conserve heat loss. Alternatively if the core temperature starts to rise the hypothalamus initiates heat loss mechanisms. A number of neurochemicals or neurotransmitters (see Ch. 5) influence the hypothalamus. Some substances including catecholamines (adrenaline, noradrenaline and dopamine) are thought to induce heat loss whilst others such as serotonin activate heat production (Mackowiak 1998). Since serotonin appears to have a significant role in thermoregulation, any disturbance in this mechanism would presumably affect the ability to maintain core body temperature within a homeostatic range. Ecstasy, an illicit drug, has attracted huge attention in the media with its association with hyperthermia. The drug seems to interfere with serotonergic neurons involved in thermoregulation and predisposes the user to hyperthermia (Milroy et al 1996). Hyperthermia is an unregulated rise in core body temperature due to a failure of the usual homeostatic mechanisms (Mackowiak 1998).

Effector mechanisms: heat loss and heat conservation

The processes by which physiological functions are adjusted to adapt to changes and maintain homeostasis are known as effector mechanisms. These effector mechanisms principally involve the sweat glands and blood vessels in the skin together with skeletal muscles.

A range of physiological and behavioural responses is promoted when the core temperature falls below the set point; some increase heat production and others conserve heat loss (Garland 1992). Heat production involves shivering, thermogenesis, and behavioural activities such as stamping feet and clapping hands together.

Cold-induced thermogenesis is heat production in response to a fall in environmental temperature; heat production results from an increase in energy expenditure. Brown adipose tissue, which is dispersed in adult humans, plays an important role in cold-induced thermogenesis. This is in response to stimulation by thyroid hormones (see Ch. 4) and sympathetic activity (see Ch. 6) (Lowell & Spiegelman 2000, Silva 2001). Thermogenesis is important in neonates (Ribeiro et al 2001), since they are unable to shiver. In newborn babies, brown adipose tissue is found in a number of locations including the adrenal glands, deep blood vessels, neck and in between the shoulder blades. This specialized adipose tissue has an abundant supply of blood vessels and mitochondria that can generate heat (Rothwell 1989).

Heat loss can be reduced by increased insulation, peripheral vasoconstriction and behavioural responses such as putting on warm clothes. In response to a decrease in core body temperature, blood flow in the skin decreases, peripheral vasoconstriction reducing the amount of blood flowing from the warm core of the body so that less heat is lost to the environment through radiation and convection. Vasoconstriction is achieved by nerve signals carried along sympathetic nerve fibres instructing smooth muscle in skin blood vessels to contract.

Following a rise in body temperature, homeostatic responses promoting heat loss and minimizing heat gains are coordinated by the hypothalamus. The major heat loss mechanisms are peripheral vasodilation and sweating. Sympathetic nerve fibres signal sweat glands to increase their activity, and sweat, a watery fluid, must then be evaporated for heat to be lost. Peripheral vasodilation is achieved as smooth muscle in the blood vessels relaxes due to decreased stimulation by sympathetic nerve impulses. This effectively means more warm blood reaches the periphery allowing heat to be lost via radiation and convection.

In summary, thermoregulation involves various heating and cooling mechanisms that are controlled by negative feedback loops. Information about temperature change is detected by peripheral and central thermoreceptors and sent to the temperature-regulating centre in the hypothalamus. This control centre instigates appropriate actions in effectors such as sweat glands and skin blood vessels to restore the core body temperature. An important feature of some homeostatic mechanisms is that behavioural responses such as putting extra clothes on when it is cold also play a key role in maintaining homeostasis.

Pyrexia

A variety of endogenous substances and drugs influence temperature regulation by modifying the activity of nerve cells in the hypothalamus (Mackowiak 1998). Fever or pyrexia, characterized by a regulated increase in core body temperature, is most commonly caused by infection and inflammation. This is why an individual's temperature is often monitored as an indicator of possible infection. There are numerous chemical substances called pyrogens which raise temperature. One important mediator of pyrexia is prostaglandin E_2 (PGE_2) secreted during the immune response. PGE_2 influences neurons within the temperature-regulating centre in the hypothalamus

to raise the temperature set point. Fever is considered an adaptive response in which the high temperature and other aspects of the febrile (fever) response have beneficial effects. There is some indication that there is a relationship between fever and an improved prognosis during infection (Kluger et al 1998, Mackowiak 1998). Despite this, pyrexia is often managed by having minimal clothing to enhance radiation, using fans to promote convection, and tepid sponging to enhance heat loss by evaporation (Watson 1998). Pyrexia is also treated by antipyretic drugs, such as aspirin, which are thought to reduce temperature by inhibiting the synthesis of PGE_2 (Aronoff & Neilson 2001).

Elective hypothermia

In contrast to accidental hypothermia, which is associated with morbidity and mortality, there are occasions when hypothermia is beneficial. In some operations the body is actively cooled. There are benefits of hypothermia in some types of surgery such as coronary artery bypass. This is because cooling the body to a core temperature of less than 34°C decreases the metabolic rate and reduces complications due to ischaemia (deficiency of blood in tissues) and reperfusion (Seekamp et al 1999).

Role of nervous and endocrine systems in homeostasis

Core body temperature is regulated mainly by the nervous system although hormones such as thyroid hormones are involved. As indicated earlier, the brain and particularly the hypothalamus are important in homeostasis. The effector mechanisms that restore homeostasis are controlled by the nervous system or by hormones. The autonomic nervous system (see Ch. 6) plays a key role; it has two divisions, the sympathetic and parasympathetic divisions, which act at an unconscious level. The sympathetic division is responsible for the 'fight and flight' response and gears the body up to respond to a challenge. It stimulates heart rate, heat production and the release of energy. Alternatively the parasympathetic nervous system is most active when we are at rest and relaxing (Rothwell 2000). A variety of hormones are also crucial in homeostasis, for example insulin, which controls blood glucose levels. Effector mechanisms controlled by hormones are usually slower in initiation and are more protracted, whilst signals carried by nerve fibres are more rapid and tend to have effects that are shorter in duration. Hormones are crucial in the homeostatic mechanisms that control blood calcium levels.

Calcium homeostasis

The homeostasis of calcium is important because calcium ions (Ca^{2+}) are crucial in a number of physiological processes including muscle contraction, blood clotting, formation of bones and teeth, cell division and neurotransmission. The principles of calcium homeostasis can be crystallized into the '3-hormone, 3-organ rule' (Rutecki & Whittier 1998). The three hormones are activated vitamin D, parathyroid hormone and calcitonin, whilst the three organs are bone, kidney and small intestine.

Bone cells

The removal (resorption) and laying down (mineralization) of bone plays a significant role in calcium homeostasis. Bone is a special form of connective tissue that is made hard, strong and durable by the addition of bone mineral, a calcium phosphate salt called hydroxyapatite. There are three types of bone cells, all of which are involved in calcium homeostasis. Osteoblasts promote mineralization or calcification in bone tissue, osteocytes are mature bone cells and osteoclasts are responsible for the resorption of bone. Osteoblasts and osteoclasts are the key protagonists in calcium homeostasis. Osteoblasts cause Ca^{2+} to be deposited in bone and lower blood Ca^{2+} levels, whilst osteoclasts cause Ca^{2+} to be released from bone and increase blood Ca^{2+} levels. The activity of these cells is controlled by parathyroid hormone (PTH) secreted from the parathyroid glands and calcitonin secreted from the thyroid gland; a number of other hormones also have an influence. PTH increases the activity of the bone resorbing osteoclasts and osteocytes, whilst calcitonin enhances the activity of osteoblasts.

Regulation of blood calcium levels is achieved by controlling the entry and exit of Ca^{2+} to and from bone. PTH also conserves calcium by enabling the kidney tubules (see Ch. 4) to reabsorb Ca^{2+} when the blood Ca^{2+} is low. PTH also stimulates the absorption of calcium from food in the small intestine by influencing the metabolism of vitamin D.

Vitamin D

Vitamin D (cholecalciferol) is a hormone rather than a vitamin. When people are exposed to enough sunlight, active vitamin D is made in the skin. Dietary vitamin D is only required when deprivation of sunlight has inhibited its activation in the skin (Mawer 1990). Many people receive vitamin D injections to treat rickets (a disease in which bones bend because they lack calcium) even though it could be easily prevented by a diet rich in calcium and exposure to sufficient sunlight (Bremer 2000). The terminology and metabolism of vitamin D is quite complicated, but in essence a prohormone in the skin, dehydrocholesterol (which as the name suggests is derived from cholesterol), is activated by sunlight to vitamin D_3 (cholecalciferol). Vitamin D_3 is released into the blood stream and carried to various organs and tissues where it is stored and/or metabolized. The main storage areas are skeletal muscle and adipose tissue and not the liver as often suggested (Mawer 1990). The vitamin becomes changed in the liver to 25-hydroxycholecalciferol and then as blood flows through the kidney it is converted, under the influence of PTH, to 1,25 dihydroxycholecalciferol, the active form of vitamin D (Mawer 1990).

Melanin

Melanin is a skin pigment that blocks out ultraviolet (UV) light and thereby reduces the risk of sunburn; it also prevents folate in the skin being broken down by UV light. So having increasing levels of melanin in the skin would seem to be beneficial. Too much melanin, however, would screen out the UV light necessary to make vitamin D_3. Skin colour could be seen as having evolved to achieve a compromise between the conflicting pressures of protecting folate in the skin and enabling sufficient vitamin D_3 synthesis to occur (Barnett 2002, Jablonski & Chaplin 2003). The two main targets for active vitamin D are the intestine where calcium is absorbed from foods and bone where calcium is laid down.

Calcitonin

Calcitonin, secreted from thyroid C cells, is another important hormone in calcium homeostasis. Calcitonin tends to lower blood calcium levels by increasing osteoblast activity, inhibiting bone resorption and encouraging urinary excretion of Ca^{2+}.

In summary, calcium homeostasis is maintained by negative feedback loops involving PTH and calcitonin. PTH tends to increase the blood calcium ion concentration when the levels are low and calcitonin tends to decrease the blood calcium ion concentration when the levels are high. Like all homeostatic loops there are three components: receptors, controllers and effectors. Receptors sensitive to calcium are found in parathyroid cells and C cells of the thyroid gland (Hory et al 1998), they are sensitive to small fluctuations in blood calcium ion concentration. The controllers are the hormones, active Vitamin D, calcitonin and PTH, and the effectors are the three organs, bone, small intestine and kidney.

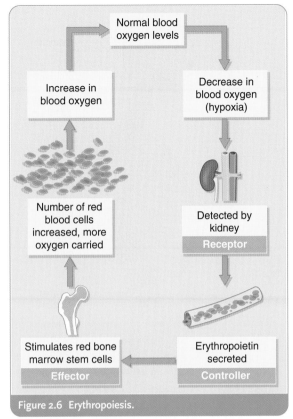

Figure 2.6 Erythropoiesis.

A hormone called erythropoietin is secreted from the kidneys when blood oxygen levels fall. Erythropoietin stimulates red bone marrow to speed up its production of red blood cells.

Erythropoiesis

Red blood cell production is a hormonally controlled homeostatic mechanism (see Fig. 2.6). Red blood cells are formed in the red bone marrow found in spongy bone. They have a limited lifespan of about 120 days because they lack a nucleus and the ability to synthesize key chemicals. A range of raw materials are needed to make a continual supply of red blood cells, which are produced at the phenomenal rate of about 2.5 million per second. These include vitamin B_{12}, folic acid, and iron to make haemoglobin, the red oxygen-carrying pigment. The rate of red blood production is controlled in a homeostatic negative feedback loop by the hormone erythropoietin.

Calcium homeostasis and erythropoiesis are two examples of homeostasis which are both linked to bone; any dysfunction in homeostasis has serious implications for health and is illustrated in a condition affecting bone called osteoporosis.

Osteoporosis

This disease is characterized by a loss of bone mass due to a reduction in the amount of calcium salts in the bones. The hormonal control of bone mineralization and bone resorption described earlier makes a significant contribution to calcium homeostasis. If this is disturbed in some way such that resorption outstrips mineralization then bone mass will decrease. An individual's bone mineral density relates to their peak bone mass (bone mass at maturity) and their subsequent bone loss with ageing. Bone remodelling increases with age and, because the rate of resorption exceeds the rate of bone formation, there is bone loss and osteoporosis (Eastell 1998). The quality of the bone also deteriorates with changes occurring in the microstructure (Watts 1999).

The consequences of loss of bone mass are that bones become increasingly fragile and prone to fracture, this is because approximately 70% of bone strength is due to its mass (Wild 1998). During their lifetime women may lose somewhere in the region of a third to a half of their skeleton (Compston 1994). Fractures are most common in the vertebrae, neck of femur and the radius. In women over 45, the main cause of hospitalization is due to fractures associated with osteoporosis (Healy 2000).

The incidence of osteoporosis increases with age and is most common in postmenopausal women, affecting one in four women (Compston 1994). In addition to PTH and calcitonin, many other hormones affect calcium homeostasis and the health of the skeletal system. These include testosterone, oestrogen, growth hormone, insulin, prostaglandins and cortisol. Deficiency of oestrogen contributes to postmenopausal osteoporosis, which has significant effects on the quality of life and results in massive healthcare costs. Oestrogen deficiency is associated with an increased number of resorption sites formed by osteoclasts together with reduced bone formation, which leads to bone loss (Compston 1994).

Osteoporosis may be prevented by building stronger bones during childhood and adolescence; women have built 98% of their skeletal mass by the age of 20 years (Bailey et al 2000). Important preventative factors are a diet rich in calcium, limited alcohol, exposure to the sun, weight-bearing exercise, no smoking and screening for signs of bone loss by testing bone density (Compston 1994, Bailey et al 2000). Vitamin D levels around the menopause also appear significant and therefore skin exposure to sunlight is important (Compston 1994).

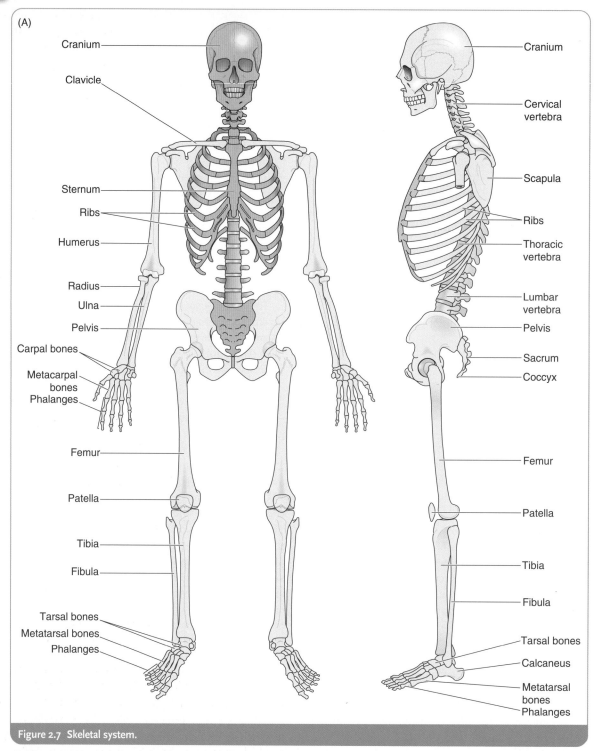

Figure 2.7 Skeletal system.

(A) The skeletal system comprises a range of bone types. (B) The long bone illustrates how form relates to function; it is hollow for lightness and strength. (C) The compact bone provides strong support relative to its weight; it contains concentric circles of bone called lamellae. (Reproduced with kind permission from Waugh & Grant 2001.)

of healthcare. Homeostasis is the basis for health and wellbeing and illness occurs when there is a failure in the mechanisms that achieve a relatively constant internal environment.

Introducing the skeletal system

The skeleton is formed from hundreds of bones linked together providing an internal framework for the body. Although there are a variety of skeletal tissues, the focus here will be on bone tissue. Bone is the hardest tissue in the body and contains living cells, water, and organic and inorganic material. Bone cells are dispersed in a matrix of inorganic salts, calcium hydroxyapatite, which make the bone rigid and hard and able to withstand compression. Collagen fibres are made of fibrous protein and form the organic part of the matrix, giving tensile strength and resilience to bone. In spite of being calcified, bone is constantly undergoing change as a result of mechanical stressors and hormones; it is dynamic rather than inert.

Bone cells and tissue

There are three types of bone cells:

- osteoblasts – responsible for creating the organic part of the matrix and its mineralization;
- osteoclasts – responsible for bone resorption and remodelling of bone due to external pressures;
- osteocytes – mature bone cells found in small spaces within the matrix (Currey 1989).

There are two types of bone tissue, compact and spongy bone, whose structure reflects their names. Compact bone is arranged in a 'compact' way, with concentric circles of bone laid around a central Haversian canal containing blood vessels, lymph vessels and nerves. The concentric circles of bone, called lamellae, contain osteocytes within small cavities called lacunae connected by a series of fine canaliculi. Canaliculi link the lacunae with the lymph vessels in the Haversian canal and provide nourishment. Haversian canals move longitudinally through bone tissue and are interconnected by transverse communicating canals, Volkman's canals, which transport nutrients and waste products (see Fig. 2.7).

Spongy, or cancellous, bone has a 'spongy' or honeycomb texture, in which the bone tissue forms a lattice of

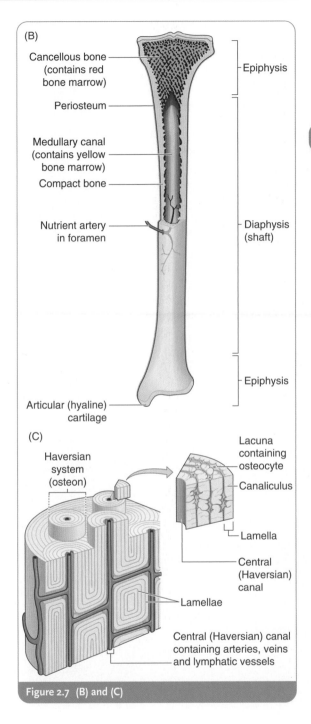

(B)

- Cancellous bone (contains red bone marrow)
- Periosteum
- Medullary canal (contains yellow bone marrow)
- Compact bone
- Nutrient artery in foramen
- Articular (hyaline) cartilage
- Epiphysis
- Diaphysis (shaft)
- Epiphysis

(C)

- Haversian system (osteon)
- Lacuna containing osteocyte
- Canaliculus
- Lamella
- Central (Haversian) canal
- Lamellae
- Central (Haversian) canal containing arteries, veins and lymphatic vessels

Figure 2.7 (B) and (C)

To conclude, osteoporosis illustrates the consequences of a breakdown in homeostasis where the two processes of bone resorption and bone mineralization are no longer properly balanced. It also illustrates how knowledge of homeostatic mechanisms should provide the rationale for the planning, delivery and evaluation

Figure 2.8 Coloured scanning electron micrograph (SEM) of human spongy bone from the shaft of a long bone.

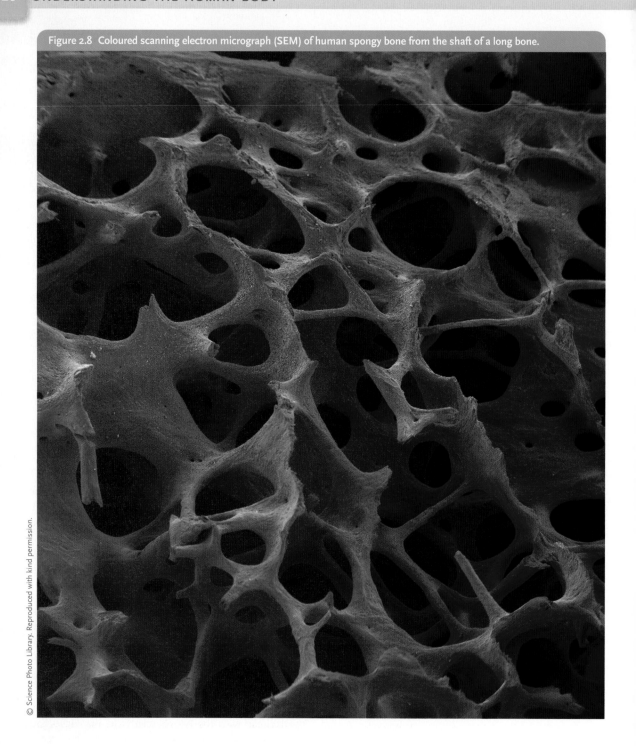

'plates and struts' (see Fig. 2.8). These consist of several lamellae containing osteocytes. The spaces in this spongy texture are filled with red bone marrow, a specialized connective tissue that contains bone marrow stem cells from which blood cells and platelets develop.

Structure of bones

The two types of bone tissue together with other tissues such as red bone marrow, adipose tissue and cartilage along with blood vessels and nerves form bones. Since bones are functional units comprised of a number of tissues, they can be classed as organs. Bones come in a variety of shapes and sizes that illustrate how form relates to function, for example, long bones (see Fig. 2.7). A long bone is a hollow structure that balances the need for lightness and strength (Currey 1989). The cylinder is made up of compact bone on the inner and outer surfaces with spongy bone sandwiched in between. The swollen ends of the long bones are called epiphyses and are specially shaped to enhance joint strength. The ends of long bones are filled with spongy bone to resist buckling. This is achieved by the network of bony struts and plates in spongy bone holding the walls of compact bone apart (Bonser 2000).

The epiphyses are covered with a special kind of cartilage, hyaline cartilage, which reduces friction in the joints and protects the bone. The tough protective covering of the bone is the periosteum. The hollow part of the long bone, the medullary or marrow cavity, contains yellow bone marrow (adipose tissue), which is a much lighter material than bone tissue.

Skeletal functions

The skeletal system has a number of functions including offering support to the body and giving it shape, enabling movement to occur at joints with the help of attached skeletal muscles, and protecting vital organs and tissues. In addition, bones within the skeletal system play a key role in calcium homeostasis and red bone marrow produces blood cells and platelets. The skeleton has two main parts, the axial skeleton, which forms the axis of the body, includes the skull, vertebral column, sternum and ribcage, and the appendicular skeleton, which consists of the limbs and limb girdles. The legs are attached to the pelvic girdle or pelvis and the arms are connected to the pectoral girdle.

References

Aronoff D M, Neilson E G 2001 Antipyretics: mechanism of action and clinical use in fever. American Journal of Medicine 111(4):304–315

Bailey K, Combs M C, Rogers L J, Stanley K L 2000 Measuring up: could this simple nursing intervention help prevent osteoporosis? AWHONN Lifelines 4(2):41–44

Barnett A 2002 Fair enough. New Scientist 176(2364):34–37

Blackburn E 1994 Prevention of hypothermia during anaesthesia. British Journal of Theatre Nursing 4(8):9–14

Bonser R 2000 Why are bones like skis? Biological Sciences Review 12(3):25–27

Bremer Z 2000 Under the sun. Nursing Standard 15(9):20

Buchman T 1996 Physiologic stability and physiologic state. Journal of Trauma 41(4):599–605

Compston J 1994 Osteoporosis: new research for old bones. MRC News 64:36–39

Currey J 1989 'Dem bones', dem bones! Biological Sciences Review 2(1):25–29

Dunbar A 1996 Altered presentation of illness in old age. Nursing Standard 10(44):49–52, 55–56

Eastell R 1998 Drug therapy: treatment of postmenopausal osteoporosis. New England Journal of Medicine 338(11):736–746

Enwright A, Plowes D 1999 Inadvertent hypothermia: is it just a perioperative problem? Nursing Standard 14(4):46–47

Garland H 1992 Homeostasis. Biological Sciences Review 4(5):12–14

Healy P 2000 Bone of contention. Nursing Standard 14(148):11

Hory B, Roussane M C, Drueke T B, Bourdeay A 1998 The calcium receptor in health and disease. Experimental Nephrology 6(3):171–179

Jablonski N G, Chaplin G 2003 Skin deep. Scientific American (Special edition) 13(2):72–79

Kaptchuk T, Croucher M 1986 The healing arts. BBC, London

Kluger M J, Kozak W, Conn C A et al 1998 Role of fever in disease. Annals of the New York Acadamy of Science 856: 224–233

Lowell B B, Speigelman B 2000 Towards a molecular understanding of adaptive thermogenesis. Nature 404(6778):652–660

Mackowiak P A 1998 Concepts of fever. Archives of Internal Medicine 158(17):1870–1881

Mackowiak P A, Boulant J A 1996 Fevers glass ceiling. Clinical Infectious Diseases 22:525–536

Mawer B 1990 The sunshine vitamin. Biological Sciences Review 2(3):2–7

McVicar A, Clancy J 1998 Homeostasis: a framework for integrating the life sciences. British Journal of Nursing 7(10):601–607

Milroy C M, Clark J C, Forrest A R W 1996 Pathology of deaths associated with 'ecstasy' and 'eve' misuse. Journal of Clinical Pathology 49(2):149–153

Porter R 1997 The greatest benefit to mankind. Harper Collins, London, p 39

Ribeiro M O, Carvalho S D, Schultz J J et al 2001 Thyroid hormone-sympathetic interaction and adaptive thermogenesis are thyroid hormone receptor isoform-specific. Journal of Clinical Investigation 108(1):97–105

Rinomhota A S, Cooper K 1996 Homeostasis: restoring the internal well being in patients/clients. British Journal of Nursing 5(18):1100–1107

Rothwell N 1989 Brown fat. Biological Sciences Review 1(4):11–14

Rothwell N 2000 Homeostasis. Biological Sciences Review 12(5): 2–5

Rutecki G W, Whittier F C 1998 Recognising hypercalcaemia: the '3-hormone, 3-organ rule': uncovering clinically important abnormalities in calcium metabolism. Journal of Critical Illness 13(1):59–66

Seekamp A, van Griensven M, Hildebrandt F et al 1999 Adenosine-triphosphate in trauma related and elective hypothermia. Journal of Trauma 47(4):673–683

Silva J 2001 The multiple contributions of thyroid hormone to heat production. Journal of Clinical Investigation 108(1):35–37

Wallis R 1994 Platelets, clots and thrombosis. Biological Sciences Review 7(2):2–6

Watts N B 1999 Focus on primary care: postmenopausal osteoporosis. Obstetrical & Gynecological Survey 54(8): 532–538

Watson R 1998 Controlling body temperature in adults. Nursing Standard 12(20):49–55

Waugh A, Grant A 2001 Ross and Wilson: Anatomy and physiology in health and illness. Churchill Livingstone, Edinburgh

Wild R 1998 Risk factors: assessment and preventative measures. Clinical Obstetrics and Gynecology 41(4):966–975

3

PROTEINS

The food that we eat provides all the chemicals that are necessary for cell structures, cell metabolism and body fluids. The principal components of cells are carbohydrates, proteins, fats and nucleic acids; we are, literally, what we eat. About 15% of the body's mass is protein, most of it in skeletal muscles. Proteins assume great importance and are the focus of this chapter because they are the chemical basis of life. No other group of molecules displays such a range of functions. They are the main building material of living organisms and are involved in regulating chemical reactions, controlling certain homeostatic mechanisms, defending against invading organisms, transporting substances around the body, and a myriad of other specialist activities (Campbell 1990). A number of important proteins will be introduced in this chapter to illustrate their strategic importance.

Proteins are macromolecules that are made from only 20 different amino acids (Bulleid 2001). Each type of protein has a different structure based on the sequence of amino acids linked together in a polypeptide chain. The sequence is dictated by genes, which contain a 'code' or set of instructions for making identical molecules of a particular protein (Bulleid 2001). Originally the human genome was considered to have about 100,000 genes, implying that there were about 100,000 different proteins responsible for human growth, development and existence (Bulleid 2001). However, the human genome project has revealed there are rather fewer human genes, somewhere in the region of 35,000 (Middleton & Peters 2001). Since each gene codes for a protein or polypeptide the number of proteins necessary for human life could be in the region of 35,000. It is more complex than this, however, because the templates formed from the gene can be modified and sections of the template can be removed. Each time this happens, a new protein is built. So there are likely to be many more proteins than there are genes in the human genome (Cohen 2000). Genes and their influence on health are discussed in detail in Chapter 10.

Some proteins are fibrous, made up of components that assemble to form insoluble fibrous structures; these include collagen, elastin and keratin, important structural proteins. Other proteins are globular, such as antibodies, plasma proteins, hormones, enzymes and haemoglobin. Globular proteins usually have a relatively compact oval or spherical shape and are soluble.

Making proteins

Cells must be able to make proteins in order to remain healthy; the cell organelle responsible for making proteins, the ribosome, was introduced in Chapter 1. The site of protein synthesis is in the cytoplasm whilst the genes containing instructions for making proteins are in the nucleus; this means that the instructions have to get to the ribosomes. This problem is solved by a copy of the DNA, in the form of a messenger RNA molecule (mRNA), leaving the nucleus. This enables the DNA template to remain safely intact within the nucleus. The analogy is taking a photocopy of an important document and keeping the original safely filed away for future use. Once in the cytoplasm the mRNA molecule becomes associated with ribosomes. The ribosomes read the message in the messenger RNA and 'translate' this information into the sequence of amino acids for that particular protein (Bulleid 2001). Protein synthesis is discussed in more detail in Chapter 10.

The copying of the DNA sequence to mRNA is called transcription and the conversion of instructions in the mRNA sequence to build the amino acid sequence by ribosomes is called translation. This chain of amino acids, a polypeptide, has to fold up into the correct three-dimensional shape. This is achieved with the help of special proteins called chaperone proteins, which guide and mould the protein (Bulleid 2001). Proteins that are destined for secretion are processed in the rough endoplasmic reticulum and sent to the Golgi body for sorting and transport out of the cell.

That protein synthesis is essential to life is illustrated by the ability of antibiotics to inhibit bacterial growth. Antibiotics have different mechanisms of action, with some being therapeutically effective because they inhibit protein synthesis. Bacteria are single-celled organisms that are different to animal cells in a number of ways, including the way in which they make proteins.

Antibiotics such as tetracycline, streptomycin, chloramphenicol and erythromycin inhibit protein synthesis in bacteria, but not human cells, and therefore can be used to treat bacterial infections without harming human cells (Franklin 1990). These antibiotics bind to bacterial ribosomes making them ineffective in synthesizing proteins, and without the proteins, the bacteria die (Bulleid 1992).

Three-dimensional shape of proteins

The construction of the polypeptide chain, with amino acids linked up in the correct sequence, is really just the first step in protein synthesis; the polypeptide then has to fold up into the right shape. The shape of proteins is crucial to their function; proteins come in all shapes and sizes and are sensitive to their environment. If proteins are denatured by a change in pH or temperature, their shape changes and their functions are lost. This is why homeostasis, discussed in Chapter 2, is so crucial; the relatively constant conditions enable proteins to maintain their appropriate shape and functions.

The structure of proteins can be described at three levels. The polypeptide chain is the primary structure or first level of protein structure. Weak attractive forces called hydrogen bonds make the chain fold up into its secondary structure. The delicate tertiary structure, which is the characteristic shape of the protein, results from other intra-molecular forces and is dictated by the sequence of amino acids in the primary structure (Brass 1995). An important feature of proteins is that many of them have distinct sections within them called 'domains'. Different domain structures are associated with different functions and shapes. The number of different domains is estimated to be somewhere between 1000–2000, which given the vast range of proteins seems remarkably small. However, different domains can be fitted together in a variety of ways and elaborated further to make the extensive range of structures and functions demonstrated by proteins (Brass 1995).

Some important proteins

Antibodies

The structure of antibodies illustrates the role of domains in shaping protein molecules. These protein molecules are present in blood and other body fluids and play a key role in immune responses. There are many different antibodies since each is specific for a different antigen. An antigen is a substance that stimulates the production of antibodies, for example, proteins found in viruses and bacteria. All antibodies have a similar structure in which characteristic domains are present, but each of them also has a unique special structure (Campbell 1990).

Specific antibodies are produced to neutralize particular antigens during an immune response. Antibodies are special proteins called immunoglobulins, and consist of four polypeptide chains arranged in a Y shape. Each antibody has subtle differences that are crucial in their defensive role (Brass 1995).

Immunoglobulins are composed of two identical heavy polypeptide chains and two identical light polypeptide chains (see Fig. 3.1). Each particular immunoglobulin has two unique binding sites; although much of the polypeptide chains are constant from one antibody to another, near the binding region there are variable regions that confer uniqueness to specific antibodies (White 1993). The antigen binds to the binding site based on matching shapes, this is sometimes described as the 'lock and key mechanism'.

Classes of antibodies

There are five classes of immunoglobulins (Ig) which are based on variations in structure and function. The constant region is identical in antibodies of the same class, but different in each of the five classes: IgG, IgM, IgA,

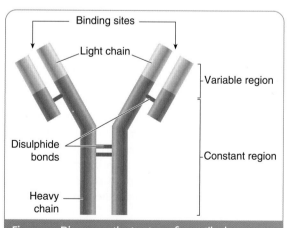

Figure 3.1 Diagrammatic structure of an antibody.

An antibody is made up of four polypeptide chains joined together to form a Y shape. The variable regions form a cleft, which acts as the antigen binding site.

IgE and IgD. Differences in their structures account for their different functions.

IgM are the largest antibodies consisting of five of these Y-shaped structures forming a pentamer; this large size restricts them to the blood stream. This structure has ten binding sites and can form many cross-links between antigen molecules causing clumps to form, a process known as agglutination. These are the first antibodies to be produced in the primary immune response, when the host meets the antigen for the first time.

> ❮ It is not difficult to deceive for the first time, for the deceived possesses no antibodies; unvaccinated by suspicion, she overlooks latenesses, accepts absurd excuses, permits the flimsiest patchings to repair great rents ... ❯
>
> (Updike 1968)

IgG antibodies are most common and are particularly important in the secondary immune response, which is stimulated on the second and subsequent exposures to a particular antigen. The secondary immune response is characterized by a swifter, greater and more sustained production of antibodies than on the first exposure to an antigen, the primary response. IgG is a single Y-shaped molecule (see Fig. 3.1); these small antibodies are present in all body fluids. Their small size enables them to cross the placenta and offer some passive immunity to the newborn baby.

IgA antibodies are found predominantly in secretions such as mucus, tears and sweat, and in digestive secretions. IgA antibodies help to protect the body from bacterial invasion by coating bacteria and preventing them from sticking to mucosal linings. They are also found in breast milk and colostrum (high-protein fluid produced prior to milk) and provide some passive immunity to the neonate. IgA molecules can link together to form dimers (two Y-shaped molecules linked together) or larger multiples.

IgD molecules are large and only found in very small amounts in blood. They are found on the surface of B-lymphocytes and are involved in recognizing antigens that the B-lymphocytes can respond to. IgE antibodies are present in very small amounts in blood and offer protection from intestinal parasites, which proliferate in unsanitary conditions in certain parts of the world. IgE also plays an important role in modulating the allergic response in conditions such as asthma (Saini & MacGlashan 2002).

Effects on antigens

Antibodies exert their effects on antigens in a number of ways, often by creating large complexes that can be eliminated. In addition to agglutination by IgM antibodies, others, notably some IgG and IgM antibodies, react with soluble antigens precipitating insoluble complexes. Another mode of action is to coat microorganisms with Ig molecules (some IgEs, IgMs and IgGs), a process called opsonization. Each of these mechanisms enhances the process of phagocytosis by specialized phagocytic cells, macrophages and neutrophils, an important feature of the immune response. Some IgM and IgG antibodies bind to the surface of bacteria and cause the cells to burst, a process called cell lysis. Finally, as already mentioned, IgA antibodies coat the surface of bacteria and stop them sticking to body surfaces, preventing them from causing infection.

Haemoglobin

Haemoglobin is a protein found in red blood cells that is able to associate with oxygen and deliver it to tissues throughout the body. There are about 280 million haemoglobin molecules in each red blood cell (Brown & Gull 1994). A haemoglobin molecule consists of four polypeptide (globin) chains and four haem groups. There are four types of globin chain with small differences in their amino acid composition, each designated by a Greek letter. Only two types of chain are present in any haemoglobin molecule. In the most common form of adult haemoglobin (HbA) there are two alpha and two beta chains. Another form of adult haemoglobin (HbA$_2$) contains two alpha and two delta chains. In the fetus, haemoglobin is specially adapted for intrauterine life, enabling effective oxygen exchange across the placenta; it is made up of two alpha and two gamma chains.

Each haemoglobin molecule consists of four subunits, each comprising of a globin chain wrapped around a haem group (see Fig. 3.2). The haem group is a complex ring structure with an iron ion at its core. Each iron ion is able to combine reversibly with an oxygen molecule, so each haemoglobin molecule can bind up to four oxygen molecules. The number of oxygen molecules that are bound to a haemoglobin molecule depends on a number of factors, including the oxygen concentration (called

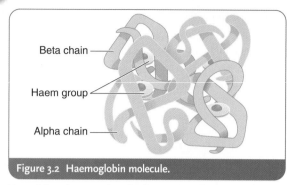

Figure 3.2 Haemoglobin molecule.

Four globin chains each with a haem group form a haemoglobin molecule. Each haem group contains an iron ion that can bind one oxygen molecule.

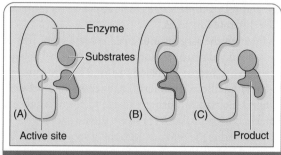

Figure 3.3 Enzyme and substrate interaction.

(A) Enzyme and substrates. (B) The substrate molecules bind to the enzyme's active site and form a temporary enzyme–substrate complex. (C) The substrate molecules are chemically changed and the product is released, leaving the enzyme unaltered and available to catalyse the same reaction again. (Reproduced with kind permission from Waugh & Grant 2001.)

partial pressure of oxygen, Po_2) surrounding the haemoglobin. When the Po_2 is high, as in the lungs, a lot of oxygen is bound, whereas in the tissues, Po_2 is low and less oxygen will be bound (Brown & Gull 1994). Therefore, haemoglobin binds oxygen in the lungs and releases it in the tissues, providing cells with oxygen necessary for survival.

The structure of the globin chains are crucial in their ability to carry oxygen. In sickle cell anaemia there is a mutation that alters just one amino acid in the beta globin chain. Sickle haemoglobin (HbS) replaces normal adult HbA in the red blood cells and this has a profound effect on the physiology and health of an individual. HbS is less efficient at carrying oxygen than HbA and it is also less soluble, which is critical since the HbS molecules change shape as Po_2 falls, forming long parallel fibres within the red blood cells. These changes cause the red blood cells to become sickle shaped; the sickle cells are less flexible and tend to form clumps that block small capillaries, leading to tissue death (Rausch & Pollard 1998). This process causes severe pain (Gorman 1999). The sickle cells have a much shorter lifespan and this leads to anaemia.

Sickle cell disease is an inherited condition and is discussed in Chapter 10. Individuals who have one HbS gene are 'carriers' and are protected from malaria infection. This protection probably led to the high frequency of HbS in individuals with an ancestry in regions of the world where malaria is or has been commonplace – such as Africa and the Mediterranean (Grant 1997). Despite this advantage, sickle cell disease is responsible for significant morbidity and mortality. This disease illustrates that the shape of a protein is crucial to function and that the concept of form related to function discussed in Chapter 1 is also applicable at the molecular level.

Enzymes

Enzymes control virtually all chemical reactions in the body. Each enzyme acts only on a particular kind of substance, called the substrate. Enzymes are the catalysts of life, speeding up chemical reactions with amazing efficiency. The shape of the enzyme molecule is crucial in its function; a slight fault will make it incapable of working. All enzymes are roughly spherical or oval shaped with a depression called the active site down one side. The shape of the substrate fits the shape of the active site. Once the active site and the substrate are joined together like two jigsaw pieces the chemical structure of the substrate is distorted, making the chemical change more likely to happen. In this way, metabolic reactions are speeded up, with rates over a million times faster (Cawston 2002). There are hundreds of different chemical reactions occurring in cells, each controlled by a specific enzyme. Enzymes are extraordinarily good at recognizing their specific substrates out of the milieu of molecules jostling about in the cell. This recognition depends upon the shape of the enzyme's active site being a perfect fit for the substrate molecule.

Enzymes catalyse chemical reactions because they overcome the energy barrier that all reactions have. The energy required for a chemical reaction to occur is called its activation energy and enzymes lower the amount of activation energy needed. When the substrate fits neatly into the active site, the substrate is held in the right position to react with other molecules. This interaction between the enzyme and its substrate has been likened to a lock and a key (see Fig. 3.3). However, a lock and key are both rigid structures whereas in reality enzyme molecules are flexible. The interaction between a substrate and its enzyme is better described as an induced fit in which the substrate causes the enzyme to change shape so that it almost envelops the substrate. The distorted enzyme puts stress on the bonds in the substrate molecule, lowering the energy barrier, and catalysis occurs. The products of the reaction are differently shaped from the substrate and diffuse away from the active site, leaving the enzyme to regain its original shape (Gull & Brown 1993, Cawston 2002).

Because the enzyme is not altered in the reaction it can be used over again. Since the shape of the enzyme is critical and enzymes, like all proteins, may be denatured, they are very sensitive to temperature change and pH, emphasizing once again the importance of homeostasis.

Certain vitamins and minerals help enzymes by making it easier for the substrate to fit into the active site. For example, vitamin C promotes the activity of enzymes involved in making collagen, a protein necessary for various connective tissues like bone and cartilage (Elliott 2002). Collagen synthesis also plays an important role in wound healing, so vitamin C is one of many nutrients essential for promoting wound healing (Truijillo 1993).

Collagen

Collagen is arguably one of the most important structural proteins in the body (Kadler 1994, Yu-Long et al 2002). It is also the most abundant protein in the body, forming the fibres of many connective tissues (Ottani et al 2002). The basic structural unit of collagen is a triple helix structure with three polypeptide chains forming a three-ply rope structure (Kadler 1994).

Collagen fibres are thick, threadlike fibres grouped together in long parallel bundles. They have some flexibility, but are relatively inelastic. Their most important attribute is that they are very strong and because of this are found in tissues and body parts holding structures together (Kadler 1994).

Collagen fibres are the main component of tendons, ligaments and the deep layer of the skin, the dermis. Collagen is also found in cartilage, bone and blood vessels. The arrangement of collagen fibres varies according to the function of the connective tissue; they are slack and flexible in the loosely woven connective tissues supporting most organs, whilst in tendons the fibres are densely packed and inelastic. The basic structure of collagen can be modified to meet the special needs of different tissues (Ottani et al 2001).

A collagen fibre comprises a bundle of parallel fibrils, slender cylindrical structures composed of even smaller microfibrils. Variations in the characteristics of a particular connective tissue can also result from differences in the collagen fibrils. Large diameter fibrils have greater tensile strength whilst smaller diameter fibrils have better 'creep resistance', meaning that they are less likely to separate as they slide past each other under stress. The arrangement of fibrils can also vary from having parallel straight molecules, as in bone, to fibrils whose molecules are helical; this type is found in a variety of tissues including skin and blood vessels (Ottani et al 2001).

That the shape of protein molecules is crucial to their function is illustrated in several collagen diseases, for example, Ehlers–Danlos syndrome. This is an inherited condition in which collagen synthesis is disturbed, leading to very long and loose collagen fibres. This causes a range of problems, including stretchy skin, loose joints and delayed wound healing (Pope & Burrows 1997).

Although collagen diseases are rare the deposition of collagen is a feature of several diseases, for example, atherosclerosis (see p. 73). In this, fatty plaques form in the lumen of arteries, stimulating inflammation, resulting in a fibrous cap composed largely of collagen fibres covering the plaque.

Collagen is not the only important structural component in skin. Bundles of collagen fibres are found in the dermis, whilst keratin (another structural protein) is located in the epidermis, the outer layer of skin. Although keratin and collagen are very insoluble and both are strong, their different functions are reflected in differences in their structure.

Keratin

Keratin forms the outer tough layer of skin, hair and nails. There are several types of keratin, but all are formed from polypeptide chains containing similar helical regions as well as other different, non-helical regions. The differences are responsible for the specific functions of keratins. Keratin chains assemble together in pairs twisting together to form a coil. Two of these two-ply structures line up together to form a four-stranded structure. The four-ply components assemble to form a keratin filament and these filaments then assemble into a lattice that contains 32 polypeptide chains (Philpott 1997). There are many different polypeptide chains. Soft keratins are found in the epidermis and hard keratins are found in nails and hair. Special skin cells called keratinocytes synthesize keratin. These cells become full of keratin and die, leaving layers of keratinized cells lying on the surface of the skin. The keratin helps to make the skin hard, tough, waterproof and a barrier to microorganisms.

Plasma proteins

Plasma contains a number of proteins, including albumins, globulins and clotting factors such as fibrinogen. The size and shape of the plasma proteins contribute to the viscosity (thickness) of the blood. Globulins include the immunoglobulins, antibodies secreted by plasma cells within the blood. The albumins and fibrinogen are made in the liver. Albumins form the largest proportion of plasma proteins and give the blood much of its osmotic pressure. The osmotic pressure of blood is important in helping to maintain its volume and pressure by attracting and holding water. Albumin forms from a single polypeptide chain of 585 amino acids (Amoresano et al 1998). Plasma proteins are also important in transporting substances in blood; for example, special globulins act as carrier proteins for thyroxine and others carry vitamins A, D and K.

Insulin

Many hormones are proteins, including growth hormone, parathyroid hormone, calcitonin and insulin. Hormones are discussed in more detail in Chapter 4, although insulin will be introduced here as a representative of the group of protein hormones that play an important role in controlling homeostasis. Insulin was the first protein to have its amino acid sequence worked out. It is a very small protein made up of only 51 amino acids in two separate chains, an A chain of 21 amino acids and a B chain of 30 amino acids, linked by disulphide bonds (Dickson 1992). Insulin is secreted from the β cells in the islets of Langerhans in the pancreas in response to raised blood glucose levels. Insulin is synthesized as a precursor pro-insulin molecule. A chain of 30 amino acids, the C-peptide, is removed from the precursor molecule during processing within the secretory vesicles. The insulin is then secreted into the blood (Kjeldsen & Andersen 1997).

Insulin has a crucial role in glucose homeostasis, a topic introduced in Chapter 2. Insulin lowers blood glucose levels by exerting a number of effects. These include stimulating uptake of glucose into cells, signalling the liver to store glucose as glycogen, inhibiting the breakdown of glycogen to glucose, and stimulating fat and protein synthesis.

In summary, proteins are extremely important molecules with diverse functions, including:

- structural proteins, such as collagen and keratin, which provide structure;
- enzymes, which control metabolic activity;
- protein hormones, such as insulin, which communicate information to cells and coordinate homeostatic mechanisms;
- haemoglobin, which carries oxygen in blood;
- antibodies, which protect us against disease.

Introducing the immune system

It is appropriate to introduce the immune system here because our immune responses rely on a range of proteins, including antibodies, cytokines, antigens, cell surface receptors and complement proteins. The human body with its relatively stable internal environment and abundant food supply is an attractive host for many bacteria, viruses, fungi and parasites. Although some of these organisms are harmless, such as certain gut bacteria introduced in Chapter 1, many cause disease. The immune system is essential for our survival; it provides resistance to infection or attack from outside the body. The first line of defence against attack, the physical barrier of skin or mucous membrane, is fairly easily overcome by disease-causing microorganisms (pathogens). Once inside the body, pathogens are first detected and then destroyed by the immune system. Another important role of the immune system is in surveillance against tumour cells.

The principal agents of destruction are the various types of white blood cells, or leucocytes. The immune system is made up of a collection of lymphoid organs and tissues, some of which are also components of other organ systems. The immune system is an effective 'defence' system because it can distinguish between 'self' and 'non-self', limit invasion of the body by pathogens, detect infected cells and recognize an infinite number of different pathogens.

The human body is equipped with a variety of defence mechanisms that prevent the entry of pathogens or destroy them following entry. Some defence mechanisms are non-specific, i.e. they protect against all pathogens, and the response is the same each time the body is exposed to an alien substance. This non-specific immunity is also called innate or inborn immunity because it is present from birth.

Other types of defence mechanisms are specific in that they provide protection against particular or specific pathogens, and only develop after exposure to that pathogen. In addition, the response on second exposure is faster and stronger than on the first encounter with the pathogen. These specific mechanisms are responsible for the individual being immune to a pathogen on a subsequent exposure.

Non-specific defences

Non-specific defences such as the skin, mucous membranes and hydrochloric acid in the stomach are relatively easily overcome by pathogens. Once inside the body antigens on the surface of pathogens are recognized by cells of the immune system as unfamiliar, 'non-self' molecules (Davey 1993). Non-specific mechanisms, phagocytosis and inflammation act quickly to destroy pathogens that have breached the mechanical and chemical barriers.

Phagocytosis

Phagocytosis is the ingestion and destruction of pathogens or other small particles, and was introduced in Chapter 1. Many cells exhibit the capacity to phagocytose, but the most important are neutrophils and macrophages. Macrophages engulf ageing cells and damaged cells as well as invading pathogens. The process of phagocytosis involves recognition, attachment and engulfment. Once inside the phagocytic cell, lysosomal enzymes digest the bacterium. As well as destroying the pathogens, macrophages digest the pathogen macromolecules into small fragments called epitopes which are held on the surface of the macrophage. The macrophage then becomes known as an antigen-presenting cell, which stimulates the specific immune defences.

Inflammatory response

Inflammation is a defensive response to tissue damage that aims to destroy pathogens and damaged cells and re-establish homeostasis. As a result of tissue trauma, chemical mediators such as histamine, serotonin and prostaglandins are released from injured cells. These chemicals have numerous effects, including dilating blood vessels to increase blood flow to the infected area. Capillary permeability increases, allowing white blood cells to leave the capillaries and enter the infected area. The increased blood flow brings more heat, making the body defences more active. Phagocytes are activated and pathogens are removed by phagocytosis.

The complement system also contributes to inflammation. This is a collection of plasma proteins activated in the immune response. Complement proteins have many roles, including the lysis of infected cells and bacteria. Complement activation is a cascade reaction similar to that of blood clotting. The cascade incorporates about 30 complement proteins whose main function is to elicit an inflammatory reaction (Nordang et al 1998).

Specific immune response

Unlike non-specific defence mechanisms, the specific immune response offers no immediate protection on the first occasion the host meets a particular antigen (primary response), but is effective on second and subsequent exposures (secondary response). The specific immune response relies on the actions of lymphocytes. These are a type of leucocyte that move around the body between the blood, tissue and lymphatic system. This re-circulation of lymphocytes ensures that they have a very good chance of meeting foreign substances. There are two types of lymphocyte, both of which originate in the bone marrow and develop from stem cells. T-lymphocytes (see Fig. 3.4) mature in the thymus gland and are responsible for cell-mediated immunity, which is particularly directed against transplanted cells, tumour cells and virally infected cells. B-lymphocytes mature in bone marrow and are responsible for humoral immunity, which is particularly directed against bacterial infections.

Humoral immune response

The humoral immune system is concerned with the production of antibodies, which as described earlier in this chapter are circulating proteins. When B-lymphocytes are stimulated by an antigen or, more accurately, when they meet an antigen presenting cell-bearing epitopes, they develop into plasma cells that secrete antibodies specific to that antigen (see Fig. 3.5). An antigen is a substance capable of promoting a specific immune response either by reacting with antibodies in humoral immunity or T-lymphocytes in the cell-mediated immune response. In reality it is the fragments of antigens, the epitopes produced by phagocytic activity of macrophages that promote these responses.

Each B-lymphocyte has the capacity to produce large quantities of its own unique antibody when needed. A particular antigen is recognized by a lock and key mechanism involving surface immunoglobulins on B-lymphocytes. Following binding, the B-lymphocyte becomes a plasma cell producing specific antibodies

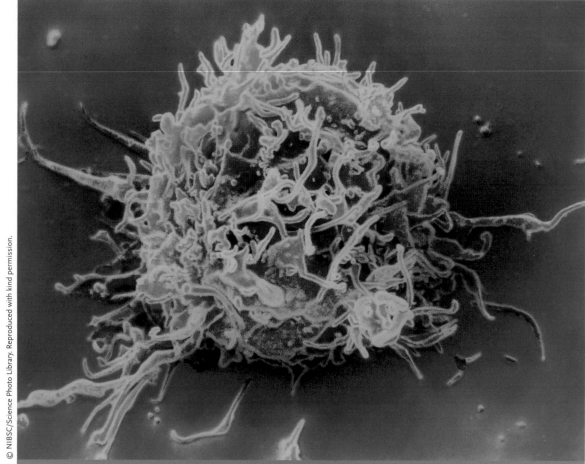

Figure 3.4 Coloured scanning electron micrograph (SEM) of a normal T-lymphocyte showing its characteristic long microvilli projecting from the cell surface.

that destroy the antigens. A clone of cells from the original B-lymphocyte remains, these are called memory cells and they elicit a swifter, magnified response in secondary immune responses.

Cell-mediated immune response

A cell-mediated immune response is initiated when an antigen binds to a specific receptor on a T-lymphocyte. In the first instance, the antigen is presented to the T-lymphocyte by an antigen-presenting cell. Once activated in this manner, T-lymphocytes undergo a series of divisions and produce groups of T-lymphocytes with different functions; all are specific to that antigen (see Fig. 3.5). Helper T-cells produce interleukins that activate other leucocytes, including lymphocytes and phagocytes. Interleukins belong to a larger group of chemicals called cytokines, proteins that enable communication between cells (Balkwill 1994). Chemicals secreted from

helper T-cells coat the phagocytes and mark them out for phagocytosis in the process called opsonization mentioned earlier (Davey 1993).

Another group of T-cells, called cytotoxic T-cells, release chemicals that ultimately puncture holes in damaged or infected cells, causing death. This activity is controlled by a further group of T-cells, the suppressor T-cells. Just as in the humoral immune response, a clone of memory cells (in this case, memory T-cells specific to the antigen) remain in circulation. On second exposure to the same antigen the cell-mediated response is greater and swifter.

The two limbs of the immune system work together during the specific immune response. Activating signals, cytokines secreted from helper T-cells, stimulate B-lymphocytes to divide, the clone of B-cells differentiate into plasma cells, which then secrete specific antibodies. Suppressor T-cells can also switch off B-lymphocytes as

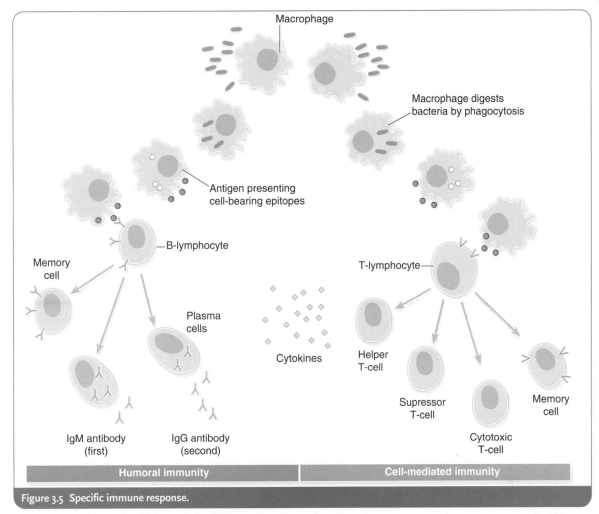

Macrophage

Macrophage digests bacteria by phagocytosis

Antigen presenting cell-bearing epitopes

B-lymphocyte

T-lymphocyte

Memory cell

Plasma cells

Cytokines

Helper T-cell

Supressor T-cell

Memory cell

IgM antibody (first)

IgG antibody (second)

Cytotoxic T-cell

Humoral immunity

Cell-mediated immunity

Figure 3.5 Specific immune response.

Macrophages engulf invading bacteria. Antigens are processed and presented as epitopes to both B-lymphocytes and T-lymphocytes. B-lymphocytes bearing specific surface immunoglobulins recognize the antigen and become plasma cells which secrete specific antibodies to that antigen. T-lymphocytes with specific receptors recognize the antigen and are stimulated to produce groups of T-lymphocytes specific to that antigen. Memory cells specific to the antigen remain in the circulation.

well as modifying the activity of other T-lymphocytes. Hence our immune responses rely on the ability of all the cells of the immune system to interact in a coordinated way (Grant 1999) and this is achieved in part by a range of proteins.

Introducing the cardiovascular system

Many different types of white blood cells have been introduced in this chapter, and whilst it has become apparent that they are not solely found in blood it is appropriate to introduce the other components of the cardiovascular system here. Blood is spun in a centrifuge into three different layers; plasma is the top layer, which amongst other substances contains the plasma proteins introduced earlier in this chapter. The middle layer contains the white blood cells and the bottom layer contains red blood cells whose form and function was introduced in Chapter 1.

In addition to transporting red and white blood cells around the body, the cardiovascular system is responsible for the rapid transport of oxygen, nutrients, waste products and heat around the body. It also contributes

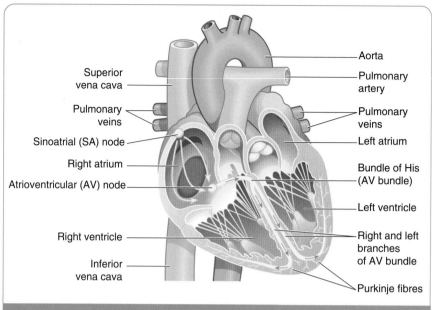

Figure 3.6 Internal structure of the heart showing the chambers and major vessels. The cardiac conduction system controls the route and timing of electrical conduction. Electrical signals travel along the pathway indicated by arrows.

to homeostasis by transporting hormones to various tissues where they exert control. The cardiovascular system comprises blood, the heart and vessels. The heart is really two muscular pumps; the right ventricle pumps blood to the lungs via the pulmonary circulation and the left ventricle pumps blood to the rest of the body via the systemic circulation.

Blood flows in a system of inter-connected vessels to tissues throughout the body. Blood leaves the heart in arteries, which then branch into smaller vessels called arterioles; in the tissues the blood enters microscopic thin-walled capillaries that enable dissolved gases, nutrients and waste products to diffuse between the capillary network and the tissues. Blood then flows back to the heart in veins, entering the heart via the venae cavae.

When the ventricles contract, a surge of blood enters the systemic arterial circulation and causes the walls of the arteries to distend, the pressure drops quickly as the contraction is completed and the elastic walls of the arteries recoil. This can be felt as the pulse at certain points where the artery runs close to the surface of the body.

The heart and cardiac conduction system

The heart has four chambers with walls of varying thickness: the left and right atria and the left and right ventricles (see Fig. 3.6). The walls of the heart have three layers: a smooth inert inner lining of squamous epithelium called the endocardium, a middle muscular layer of cardiac muscle called the myocardium and an outer fibrous layer called the pericardium.

The atria and ventricles contract in sequence. The cardiac cycle is a series of pressure and volume changes lasting for 0.9 seconds. One cardiac cycle includes systole, which is when the heart is contracting, followed by diastole, when the heart relaxes. The cardiac cycle is controlled by a special electrical system called the cardiac conduction system, which consists of specialized muscle cells located in the walls of the heart (see Fig. 3.6). The sinoatrial (SA) node initiates the heartbeat, this 'pacemaker' discharges spontaneously at regular intervals. This firing is independent of nervous input, although the rate of firing can be influenced by nerve impulses from the cardiac centre located in part of the brain stem called the medulla oblongata. Once the pacemaker discharges, a wave of depolarization spreads across the atria causing them to contract, pushing blood into the ventricles. The electrical impulse reaches the atrioventricular (AV) node and, after a short delay that enables the atria to empty completely, the electrical impulse reaches the bundle of His and its branches. The bundle fibres distribute the electrical impulse throughout the ventricular walls causing them to contract, forcing blood into the major arteries. The electrical activity of the cardiac cycle can be recorded, giving rise to ECG (electrocardiogram) waves. These can indicate normal heart activity or highlight abnormal patterns in the cardiac rhythm.

Control of heart activity

The activity of the heart is controlled so that blood is pumped around the body to match the physiological needs demanded by different levels of activity, such as

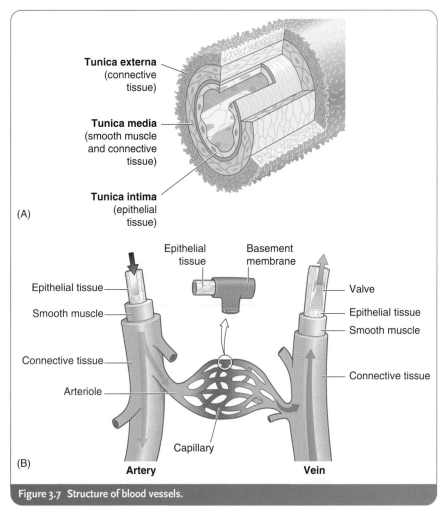

oxygen, an external control system is also required. This is achieved by the autonomic nervous system (see Ch. 6). The heart is supplied by both sympathetic and parasympathetic nerves originating in the cardiac centre in the medulla. Sympathetic fibres connect with the SA node, AV node and cardiac muscle and impulses carried along these fibres cause the secretion of noradrenaline, a neurotransmitter that increases heart rate and force of muscle contractions. Impulses transmitted along parasympathetic fibres to the SA node and AV node cause the secretion of acetylcholine at the nerve endings. Acetylcholine suppresses heart activity, causing the heart rate to slow and force of muscle contractions to decrease. Since cardiac output is directly proportional to blood pressure, controlling heart rate and stroke volume are also central to the control of blood pressure. Blood vessels also contribute to the regulation of blood pressure.

Figure 3.7 Structure of blood vessels.

(A) The three basic layers found in arteries and veins are shown. (B) The layer of smooth muscle is thicker in the artery compared to the vein. By comparison the capillary has a much thinner wall.

rest, gentle activity or strenuous exercise. The action of the heart determines how much blood enters the arterial system; if more blood is pumped out, the blood pressure will increase and vice versa. The cardiac output is the amount of blood pumped out of the heart during a minute and is calculated thus:

cardiac output = stroke volume × heart rate

where the stroke volume is the amount of blood ejected from the left ventricle at each contraction.

The heart muscle must contract in a coordinated fashion to ensure efficient pump action. This is achieved by the cardiac conduction system, which via the 'pacemaker' generates a rhythmical rate of contraction between about 70 to 100 beats per minute. Since the heart rate varies to meet the changing requirements of the tissues for

Structure and function of blood vessels

Blood is transported around the body in a network of vessels that, although similar in some respects, are adapted to their particular functions (see Fig. 3.7). Both arteries and veins have a similar structure, made up of three basic layers. The inner layer, or tunica intima, is a single layer of squamous epithelium called endothelium that is supported by connective tissue containing elastic fibres. This provides a smooth surface allowing blood cells to flow through without damage. The elasticity enables the vessel to stretch and accommodate blood flowing through it. The middle layer, or tunica media, is composed of smooth muscle and elastic connective tissue. The smooth muscle is supplied with sympathetic nerve fibres that can alter the diameter of the vessel.

Changes in diameter are crucial in altering the flow and pressure of blood. The outer layer, or tunica externa, is a layer of connective tissue containing elastic and collagen fibres that protects the vessel. The relative thickness and composition of each layer varies depending on the vessel's function. The middle layer shows the greatest variation.

Capillaries are comprised solely of the inner layer described above; their walls consist of endothelium, a single layer of squamous epithelium through which substances can diffuse in and out.

Control of blood pressure

Blood pressure is carefully controlled to match changing physiological needs so that homeostasis is maintained. Blood pressure in arteries rises and falls in a pattern that relates to the phases of the cardiac cycle. The pressure is highest during ventricular systole (contraction) and lowest during ventricular diastole (relaxation).

Blood pressure control is achieved by a number of homeostatic mechanisms, including the control exerted by the cardiac centre over heart activity. In addition, another group of neurons in the medulla, the vasomotor centre, regulates the diameter of arterioles. This is an important aspect of blood pressure regulation since the pressure of blood increases if it is forced through a narrower vessel. The force created by the friction between blood and the walls of blood vessels is called peripheral resistance. The greater the peripheral resistance, the higher the blood pressure, whilst less resistance equates to a lower blood pressure. The diameter of the arterioles is controlled by the contraction and relaxation of smooth muscle in their walls. Sympathetic fibres from the vasomotor centre carry impulses to the smooth muscle of the arteriole walls all the time. When the frequency of nerve impulses is high, smooth muscle contracts more, resulting in vasoconstriction, and when the rate of impulses is slower vasodilation occurs.

The short-term control of blood pressure is achieved by both the cardiac centre and vasomotor centre responding swiftly to information received by baroreceptors found in the aortic arch and internal carotid arteries. These pressure-sensitive receptors detect changes in blood pressure and send signals to both centres. So a fall in blood pressure, which might be caused by getting up suddenly after lying down, would be detected by baroreceptors. As a consequence these receptors send fewer impulses to both the cardiac and vasomotor centres. The cardiac centre has two regions and in response to falling blood pressure more sympathetic impulses would leave the cardioacceleratory centre and less parasympathetic impulses from the cardioinhibitory centre. This would excite the SA node, AV node and cardiac muscle resulting in an increase in heart rate and stroke volume. The increased cardiac output would raise blood pressure and restore homeostasis.

Sympathetic impulses from the vasomotor centre would also increase, causing vasoconstriction of arterioles and a resultant rise in blood pressure. Both the cardiac centre and vasomotor centre can be influenced by a variety of factors in addition to changes in blood pressure, including blood gas concentrations, temperature, pH and hormones. The hormonal control of fluid balance (see Ch. 4) contributes to blood pressure but is slower and relates to changes in blood volume.

The cardiovascular system is adapted to pump blood effectively around the body according to need. A key function of blood is to transport a variety of substances to tissues throughout the body. Important cargoes in this transport system are the numerous proteins, including plasma proteins, immunoglobulins, hormones, complement proteins and red blood cells containing the protein haemoglobin.

References

Amoresano A, Andolfo A, Siciliano R A et al 1998 Analysis of human serum albumin variants by mass spectrometric procedures. Biochimica et Biophysica Acta 1384(1):79–92

Balkwill F 1994 Cytokines. Biological Sciences Review 7(2):23–27

Brass A 1995 Protein structure. Biological Sciences Review 7(5):28–30

Brown B, Gull D 1994 Haemoglobin. Biological Sciences Review 6(3):14–16

Bulleid N 1992 How are proteins made? Biological Sciences Review 4(5):2–4

Bulleid N 2001 Tailor-made proteins. Biological Sciences Review 13(4):2–6

Campbell P 1990 Variations on a protein theme. Biological Sciences Review 2(3):15–19

Cawston T 2002 Enzymes. Biological Sciences Review 15(1):2–5

Cohen P 2000 High in protein. New Scientist 168(2263):38–41

Davey B 1993 The immune system. Biological Sciences Review 5(5):15–19

Dickson A J 1992 Insulin and diabetes. Biological Sciences Review 4(4):2–5

Elliott W L 2002 Role of vitamin C in collagen biosynthesis and connective tissue health. Biological Sciences Review 6(4):221–224

Franklin T 1990 Antibiotics: magic bullets and enchanted rings. Biological Sciences Review 2(3):26–27

Gorman K 1999 Sickle cell disease. American Journal of Nursing 99(3):38–43

Grant A 1999 Lymphocytes. Biological Sciences Review 12(1):32–35

Grant M 1997 Globins, genes and globinopathies. Biological Sciences Review 9(4):2–5

Gull D, Brown B 1993 Enzymes – fast and flexible. Biological Sciences Review 6(2):26–28

Kadler K 1994 Collagen. Biological Sciences Review 6(4):35–38

Kjeldson T, Andersen A S 1997 Insulin from yeast. Biological Sciences Review 10(2):30–32

Middleton L A, Peters K F 2001 Genes and Inheritance. Cancer Nursing 24(5):357–369

Nordang L, Laurent C, Mollnes T E 1998 Complement activation in sudden deafness. Archives of Otolaryngology – Head & Neck Surgery 124(6):633–636

Ottani V, Raspanti M, Ruggeri A 2001 Collagen structure and functional implications. Micron 32(3):251–260

Ottani V, Martini D, Franchi M et al 2002 Hierarchical structures in fibrillar collagens. Micron 33(7–8):587–596

Philpott M 1997 Keratin. Biological Sciences Review 9(3):36–38

Pope F M, Burrows N P 1997 Ehlers-Danlos syndrome has varied molecular mechanisms. Journal of Medical Genetics 34(5): 400–410

Rausch M, Pollard D 1998 Management of the patient with sickle cell disease. Journal of Intravenous Nursing 21(1):27–40

Saini S S, MacGlashan D 2002 How IgE upregulates the allergic response. Current Opinions in Immunology 14:694–697

Truijillo E B 1993 Effects of nutritional status on wound healing. Journal of Vascular Nursing 11(1):12–18

Updike J 1968 Couples. Penguin, Harmondsworth, p 131

Waugh A, Grant A 2001 Ross and Wilson: Anatomy and physiology in health and illness. Churchill Livingstone, Edinburgh

White A 1993 Antibodies. Biological Sciences Review 6(2):20–22

Yu-Long S, Zong-Ping L, Fertala A et al 2002 Direct quantification of the flexibility of type 1 collagen monomer. Biochemical and Biophysical Research Communications 295(2):382–386

4

HORMONES

‘ The emergency doctor came to my Grandma's last night at 11.30 pm. He diagnosed that I am suffering from *acne vulgaris*. He said it was so common that it is regarded as a normal state of adolescence. He thought it was highly unlikely that I have got lassa fever because I have not been to Africa this year. He told Grandma to take the disinfected sheets off the doors and windows. Grandma said she would like a second opinion. That was when the doctor lost his temper. He shouted in a very loud voice, 'The lad has only got a few teenage spots for Christ's sake!' ’

(Townsend 1982)

The word 'hormone' comes from the Greek word *hormon* which means 'to stir up'. Hormones often get blamed for mood swings in females, aggressive behaviour in males (Fausto-Sterling 1992), and the unpredictability of adolescents (McCrone 2000). In the above quotation from *The Secret Diary of Adrian Mole aged 13¾* there is an implicit link between adolescence, hormones and teenage spots! A more accurate view of hormones is that they are dynamic contributors to homeostasis and health (see Ch. 2). Hormones influence all bodily functions, from the most basic to the more subtle and sublime. Hormones are highly potent chemicals that control almost all aspects of our lives including growth, development, metabolism, reproduction and our ability to cope with stress.

Hormones are chemical messengers secreted by endocrine glands or, in some cases, endocrine tissues. Endocrine hormones are secreted directly into blood. The tissues that the hormone exerts its effects on are called target tissues and are traditionally described as being distant to the endocrine gland secreting the hormone. However, chemical messengers can communicate in different ways. Some hormones, like prostaglandins, are secreted into tissue fluid and have effects on neighbouring cells, this is called paracrine communication. Because prostaglandins act locally they are sometimes described as 'local hormones'. Autocrine communication is when the hormones or other chemical signals secreted into the tissue fluid influence the activity of the cell that originally secreted them.

Whilst this chapter is focused on hormones, there are other chemical messengers, including neurotransmitters (see Ch. 5) and pheromones, that are released out of the body and carry information to other members of the same species. Pheromones are sometimes described as 'volatile hormones' (Debuse 1998). Pheromones are thought to trigger responses such as sexual arousal and

defensive behaviour in many species. Some animals have a special organ called a vomeronasal organ (VNO) that responds to these pheromonal cues by signalling information to the hypothalamus, the part of the brain involved in feeding, reproduction and fighting. There is evidence for a VNO in human fetuses, but the existence of a functioning VNO in adult humans is much more controversial (Taylor 1997, Keverne 1999, Firestein 2001). The idea that humans might also communicate via pheromones is contested. Women living together often synchronize their menstrual cycles, but whether this is as a result of pheromone signalling is still not clear (Weller 1998). Another interesting aspect of chemical signals and reproductive behaviour is the possibility that humans might choose their partners based on their smell (Small 1999). Preferences for body odours of potential mates might be connected with their genetic appropriateness. Genetic difference in a mate is important and this 'difference' seems to be centred on a group of genes that are key to immune responses (Motluk 2001).

Hormonal chemistry

Hormones coordinate functions and enable communication within the body rather than between bodies. The way in which hormones interact with target cells depends on their chemistry. Although there are a number of different categories of hormones, including peptides, proteins, amino acid derivatives, steroids and prostaglandins, most hormones, with exceptions such as prostaglandins, belong to one of two main groups. Hormones synthesized from amino acids, including proteins, peptides and amino acid derivatives, interact with cell surface receptors, whilst steroid hormones interact with cytoplasmic or intracellular receptors. Target cells possess thousands of receptor proteins for the hormones they respond to. Many cells also have receptors for neurotransmitters so they can be influenced by both types of signalling molecules.

Protein, peptide and amino acid derived hormones are soluble in water, but only slightly soluble in lipid. This means the hormones cannot diffuse into the cell across the fatty cell membrane, but require special receptors in the cell membrane to bind with. The following are examples of polypeptide and protein hormones:

- insulin and glucagon – regulate blood glucose levels;
- antidiuretic hormone – helps to maintain fluid balance;
- prolactin – controls milk production.

The following are examples of hormones derived from amino acids:

- adrenaline and noradrenaline – involved in the alarm response;
- thyroid hormones – regulate growth and metabolism.

Steroid hormones are synthesized from cholesterol and are lipid soluble. This means that they can readily diffuse across the fatty plasma membrane into target cells and interact with intracellular hormone receptors (Tsai & O'Malley 1994). All steroids have a similar chemical structure and, because of this, their roles may overlap. The following are examples of steroid hormones:

- oestrogen, progesterone and testosterone – regulate reproductive functions;
- aldosterone – regulates sodium balance;
- cortisol – influences metabolism and promotes response to stress (see Ch. 6).

Prostaglandins, derived from fatty acids in the cell membrane, are produced by most cells in the body. Prostaglandins have both autocrine and paracrine effects and are involved in numerous activities, including mediating the inflammatory and pain responses, and in vasodilation. They are also implicated in fever (Funk 2001). Prostaglandins belong with leukotrienes, which also act locally and are produced from fatty acids, in a class of hormones called eicosanoids (Baxter & Ribeiro 2001).

Mechanism of hormone action

Hormones are effective in very small amounts, only a few molecules are needed to stimulate a dramatic response. There are many variations in the way hormones act on their target cells; some, for example adrenaline, have a rapid action whereas others, for example oestrogen, are slower in their effects. The function of hormones is to modify the physiological activity of target cells and they do this by regulating the activity of cell enzymes or by controlling the entry of substances into the cell. Hormones that bind to cell surface receptors usually elicit a rapid response whilst steroid hormones tend to produce a slow sustained response (Westwood 1999).

Hormones interacting with cell-surface receptors

Hormones synthesized from amino acids bind to specific receptors on the cell membrane (see Fig. 4.1). These receptors are proteins embedded within the phospholipid bilayer of the plasma membrane. Following binding, the hormone receptor complex activates chemicals which are referred to as second messengers, the first messenger being the hormone itself. Target cells generate one of several types of second messenger in response to hormone interaction, including cyclic adenosine monophosphate (cAMP), cyclic guanosine monophosphate (cGMP), calcium ions and various modified membrane lipids. These second messenger molecules activate enzymes called protein kinases that lead to activation of further enzymes in a cascade reaction. In this way, one hormone molecule can lead to the activation of hundreds of enzyme molecules.

Receptors that lead to the generation of second messenger molecules are linked to G proteins in the plasma membrane. G proteins play a crucial part in the cascade system, which amplifies the cell response to a hormone. Once the target cell has responded to the hormone, the second messenger molecules are deactivated (Gardner 2001).

The mechanism of action of prostaglandins is still being investigated, but most seem to interact with receptors in the cell membrane in a similar fashion to many peptide and protein hormones. Prostaglandin receptors are linked to G proteins that generate second messengers (Funk 2001).

Steroid hormones interacting with intracellular receptors

Steroid hormones are lipid soluble and can easily diffuse across the cell membrane and interact with

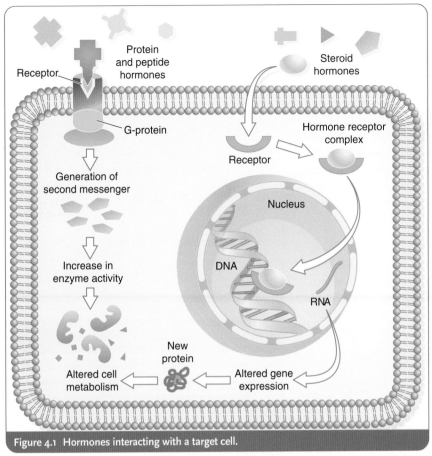

Figure 4.1 Hormones interacting with a target cell.

Protein and peptide hormones (first messengers) bind with hormone receptors in the plasma membrane of target cells. This ultimately leads to the generation of a second messenger, which activates specific intracellular enzymes. The activated enzymes lead to a change in cell metabolism. Steroid hormones interact with intracellular receptors. The hormone receptor complex enters the nucleus and binds to a specific site on a DNA molecule. This switches on a gene and initiates protein synthesis. This new protein is often an enzyme which alters cell metabolism.

are diverse. Secretion from some endocrine glands is stimulated by nerve impulses, for example, the secretion of adrenaline from the adrenal medulla is controlled by sympathetic nerve impulses. Stressors such as pain, exercise and fear will lead, via sympathetic fibres, to bursts of adrenaline being secreted. The activity of several endocrine glands, the testes, ovaries, thyroid gland and adrenal cortex, is controlled by hormones from the hypothalamus and anterior pituitary gland. Finally, the secretion of other hormones is controlled by changes in a variable monitored in body fluids; for example, changes in blood glucose levels stimulate the secretion of insulin or glucagon.

Many hormones show fluctuations that are rhythmic. These hormonal rhythms are important for general wellbeing and health. Some hormones show high and low peaks occurring every few minutes or hours; for example, luteinizing hormone is secreted every 90–120 minutes (Griffiths 1993). Other hormones such as cortisol fluctuate over a 24-hour cycle, while others such as follicle-stimulating hormone and oestrogen involved in the menstrual cycle ebb and flow on a monthly basis (see p. 122).

The hypothalamus and pituitary gland are the main coordinators of the endocrine system since between them they secrete a range of hormones that regulate the activity of several other endocrine glands.

specific receptors in the cytoplasm (see Fig. 4.1). Following hormone receptor binding, the hormone receptor complex enters the nucleus of the target cell and binds to DNA. This 'switches on' particular genes and leads to the production of mRNA and ultimately protein synthesis (see p. 129). Some of the proteins manufactured will be enzymes that alter the cell's metabolic activity.

Regulation of hormone activity

Since hormones are messengers they are not secreted continuously, but only in the right amounts to maintain homeostasis. The stimuli for the release of hormones

Hypothalamus and pituitary gland

One of the reasons the hypothalamus is able to play such a key role in homeostasis is that it is connected to many parts of the nervous system by nerve fibres. The hypothalamus links the mind and body (see Ch. 6) and because it controls the pituitary gland it can exert influence on all cells in the body.

The pituitary gland lies immediately below the hypothalamus at the base of the brain; it has two parts, the anterior pituitary gland (adenohypophysis) and the posterior pituitary gland (neurohypophysis). The hypothalamus secretes a number of releasing and inhibitory hormones that control the activity of various endocrine cells in the anterior pituitary gland. Both parts of the pituitary gland connect to the hypothalamus; the anterior pituitary gland is linked via a blood supply whilst the posterior pituitary gland is connected via nerve tracts. Hypothalamic hormones travel via blood to the anterior pituitary gland and via nerve fibres to the posterior pituitary gland.

The anterior pituitary gland responds to hypothalamic hormones by altering its secretion of a number of hormones. Several anterior pituitary hormones are responsible for controlling the activity of other endocrine glands. Between them, therefore, the hypothalamus and anterior pituitary gland orchestrate a wide range of hormonal responses.

Anterior pituitary gland

A variety of hormones that have direct effects on target cells are secreted by different types of endocrine cells in the anterior pituitary gland. These include growth hormone, prolactin and melanocyte-stimulating hormone. The latter increases skin pigmentation by stimulating accumulation of melanin in melanocytes, skin cells found under the epidermis. Other hormones act indirectly by controlling the activity of certain endocrine glands. These hormones are described as trophic or stimulating hormones and control the activity of target endocrine glands: the thyroid gland, adrenal cortex, ovaries and testes (gonads).

Therefore there is an axis of control in these four endocrine glands (see Fig. 4.2). Within this hierarchy of control, negative feedback systems operate; when the hormones secreted from the target endocrine gland reach critical levels, they inhibit the activity of certain endocrine cells in both the hypothalamus and the anterior pituitary gland. This means that less hypothalamic releasing hormone and less stimulating hormone from the anterior pituitary will be secreted. As a consequence hormone secretion from the target endocrine gland decreases. When the level of this hormone falls, the inhibition on the hypothalamus and anterior pituitary gland will lift. These feedback loops enable hormone secretion to be controlled with precision.

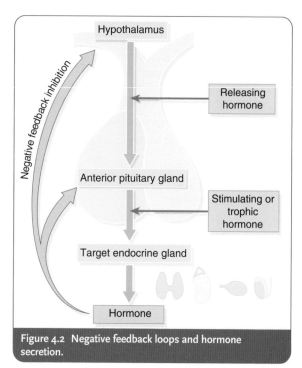

Figure 4.2 Negative feedback loops and hormone secretion.

The secretion of hormones from the ovaries, testes, thyroid gland and adrenal cortex is regulated by negative feedback loops involving the hypothalamus and anterior pituitary gland.

Posterior pituitary gland

This gland releases oxytocin and antidiuretic hormone, which are made in specialized hypothalamic neurons. These hormones travel along the nerve fibres into the posterior lobe of the pituitary gland where they are stored. Nerve impulses from the hypothalamus signal the posterior pituitary gland to release its hormones. Antidiuretic hormone (ADH) and oxytocin are very similar in structure; both are peptide hormones consisting of a chain of nine amino acids. There is some overlap in their functions, both have an antidiuretic action and both cause smooth muscle contraction. The principal role of ADH is in water conservation and maintaining fluid balance. Oxytocin's main function is to cause smooth muscle contraction of the uterus and contraction of specialized myoepithelial cells in breast tissue, which allows milk to flow during breast feeding.

Many hormones that are engaged in control, communication and integration have already been mentioned. The control of metabolic rate and fluid and electrolyte balance will now be explored to illustrate the roles of several hormones in more detail.

Control of metabolic rate

All hormones contribute to metabolism to some extent, but certain hormones, such as the thyroid hormones, have a major role in the regulation of metabolism and the rate at which energy is used in the body. The thyroid gland is a butterfly-shaped organ at the base of the neck that secretes two thyroid hormones, thyroxine, which is produced in the largest amounts, and tri-iodothyronine, which is more potent. Both hormones are not only involved in increasing the metabolic rate, but also in the growth and development of the skeletal system, temperature regulation and reactivity of the nervous system. Another hormone, calcitonin, involved in calcium homeostasis (see Ch. 2), is also secreted from the thyroid gland, but from a different group of cells, called C cells.

The thyroid gland needs iodine to function properly: thyroxine has four atoms of iodine and is known as T_4 and tri-iodothyronine contains three iodine atoms and is called T_3. Both hormones are derived from the amino acid, tyrosine (McPherson 2000), to which iodine is added. The cells of the thyroid gland are able to transfer iodine from the blood and concentrate it. If there is a lack of iodine in the diet, the thyroid gland enlarges and a goitre develops. Iodine is added to salt to ensure there are sufficient amounts in the diet to prevent goitres. The ability of the thyroid gland to concentrate iodine is capitalized on in the adjuvant treatment of thyroid cancer; radioactive iodine is used because it has a localized effect on the thyroid gland (Sherman 2003).

The thyroid gland is made up of secretory units called follicles. Follicles are hollow spheres, containing thyroglobulin, a complex protein stored within a thick fluid called colloid. This is surrounded by a follicular wall composed of cuboidal epithelial cells. These follicle cells synthesize both T_3 and T_4 thyroid hormones and thyroglobulin. Thyroglobulin stores the excess thyroid hormones, which can be released by enzymes when the hormones are required. The hormones diffuse into the blood, bind to plasma proteins and are carried to their target cells. T_3 and T_4 hormones, unlike other amino acid derived hormones, interact with intracellular receptors rather than cell surface receptors. The hormones bind to receptors and stimulate protein synthesis and an increased production of cell enzymes (Tsai & O'Malley 1994), which ultimately increases metabolism.

When the metabolic rate is too low, special cells in the hypothalamus detect the decreased levels of thyroid hormones in the blood. In response, the hypothalamus secretes thyrotropin-releasing hormone (TRH) into the blood. This stimulates the anterior pituitary gland to release thyroid-stimulating hormone (TSH) also known as thyrotropin. This hormone in turn increases the activity of the follicle cells. T_3 and T_4 hormones are released into the blood and the metabolic rate is restored to appropriate levels. This is a good illustration of negative feedback (see Fig. 4.2). Whilst the metabolic rate usually is maintained within normal limits, it can be modified to respond to environmental and emotional triggers such as temperature, exercise, eating, anxiety and depression.

Fluid and electrolyte balance

In homeostasis and health, the volume of fluid in our bodies and the concentration of electrolytes in body fluids are regulated by balancing the intake of water and electrolytes against all losses. Fluid output includes what is excreted in urine, or lost from the lungs as we breathe or via the surface of the body in sweat. Both fluid input and fluid output are regulated. We feel thirsty if the volume of fluid falls and this stimulates us to have a drink. At the same time fluid output is adjusted by producing variable amounts of urine to achieve fluid balance. This variation in urine production is controlled by hormones acting on the nephrons, the functional units of the kidney (see p. 52). Various hormones influence fluid and electrolyte balance, but antidiuretic hormone (ADH), aldosterone and atrial natriuretic peptide (ANP) are most significant. Other hormones that affect fluid balance, but to a lesser extent, include prolactin, growth hormone and oestrogen.

Before moving on to discover how these hormones contribute to fluid and electrolyte balance you might find it useful to read the section that introduces the urinary system and the kidneys (see p. 52). The kidneys are responsible for filtering harmful substances out of blood and varying the quantities of water and ions passed out in urine to maintain fluid and electrolyte balance. Selective reabsorption of water and sodium ions occurs as the filtrate passes through the kidney tubules. Water reabsorption is controlled by ADH whilst movement of sodium ions between the tubule and surrounding blood capillaries is controlled by aldosterone and ANP.

Antidiuretic hormone

ADH (also known as vasopressin) is produced in the hypothalamus by giant nerve cells whose axons carry the hormone to the posterior pituitary gland where the hormone is stored in nerve endings (Farrar & Balment 1990). ADH is a peptide hormone that increases the reabsorption of water from the kidney tubules. In the absence of ADH the distal convoluted tubule and collecting duct are impermeable to water; ADH increases their permeability so that water passes out of the tubule and eventually into the surrounding blood capillaries. This results in a small quantity of concentrated urine being produced. The secretion of ADH is regulated by negative feedback mechanisms (see Fig. 4.3), but a variety of stimuli such as pain, anxiety and various drugs can also influence ADH secretion. Alcohol causes alteration in ADH secretion, and an alcohol hangover is associated with dehydration. This is due to alcohol

inhibiting the effect of ADH on the kidney tubules, this means less water is reabsorbed and a diuresis (increased volume of urine excreted) occurs (Wiese et al 2000).

Since ADH is a peptide, it interacts with specific cell surface receptors in its target cells and generates cAMP, a second messenger molecule. The second messenger ultimately leads to an increase in permeability of the target cells to water. Water channels in cell membranes within the kidney tubule and many other tissues are special proteins called aquaporins (Kozono et al 2002). Different kinds of aquaporins are involved in the increased permeability to water elicited by ADH. When

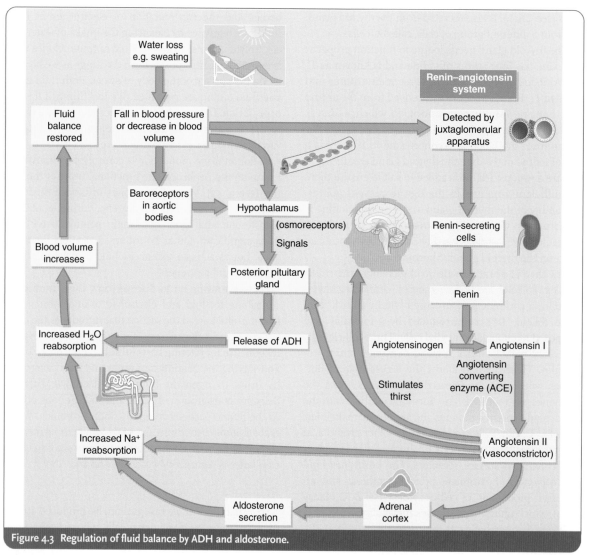

Figure 4.3 Regulation of fluid balance by ADH and aldosterone.

A decrease in fluid volume or a fall in blood pressure causes more ADH to be released from the posterior pituitary gland. ADH increases water reabsorption in the nephron. The fall in blood pressure also stimulates the renin–angiotensin–aldosterone system. Aldosterone stimulates water reabsorption in the nephron by increasing reabsorption of sodium ions (Na^+).

ADH reaches its target cells in the kidney tubules it instructs the cells to make more aquaporins, which once inserted into the plasma membrane allow more water to be reabsorbed back into the blood. When the concentration of ADH falls, the aquaporin molecules disappear and the kidney tubules become impermeable once more (Steward 1996).

The production and release of ADH is controlled by negative feedback (Farrar & Balment 1990). Specialized nerve cells in the hypothalamus have particular aquaporins in the plasma membrane, which enables the osmotic pressure of blood to be monitored. When the osmotic pressure of blood increases, less water flows into these specialized cells (called 'osmoreceptors') and they shrink. This stimulates the release of ADH from the posterior pituitary gland (Steward 1996) and also stimulates thirst and drinking behaviour (Lote 1993). The ADH travels in blood to the kidneys where it stimulates increased reabsorption of water into blood from the distal convoluted tubules and collecting ducts. The osmotic pressure of blood therefore decreases and homeostasis is maintained (see Fig. 4.3).

Urination shows a circadian rhythm with more urine being produced in the morning and less being produced at night; there may be a number of reasons for this observed pattern including variable fluid intake throughout the day, differences in glomerular filtration rate and the diurnal rhythm of ADH secretion. The increased incidence of nocturia in older people is thought to relate to a loss of this diurnal pattern (Asplund & Aberg 1991). Producing less ADH at night may cause an older person to produce more urine nocturnally (Lose et al 2001).

An important concept in hormone action is that many hormones affect neural function, sometimes directly, such as sex steroids influencing sexual behaviour, or indirectly, such as the effects of low glucose levels on mental function caused by too much insulin. Antidiuretic hormone appears to play a role in enhancing learning and memory. There are hormone receptors in the hippocampus, an area of the brain involved in memory formation. ADH interacts with these receptors at a local level within the brain and so may be considered a neuropeptide (Alescio-Lautier et al 2000).

Aldosterone secretion

Aldosterone is a hormone synthesized by the adrenal cortex. It is called a mineralocorticoid since it helps to keep the concentrations of 'mineral' electrolytes (sodium and potassium ions) in balance. Aldosterone is a steroid hormone and interacts with intracellular receptors. Although the precise mechanism remains unclear, aldosterone interaction with target cells within the distal convoluted tubule leads to an increase in epithelial sodium channels (Loffing et al 2001). Aldosterone enables its target cells to become more permeable to sodium ions, which are then reabsorbed back into blood whilst at the same time potassium ions are excreted. Since aldosterone conserves sodium ions it also causes more water to be reabsorbed because water follows the sodium ions by osmosis.

Aldosterone secretion is mainly under the control of the renin–angiotensin–aldosterone system (see p. 53). Angiotensin II is produced when there is a fall in blood pressure (see Fig. 4.3) and it promotes the release of aldosterone from the adrenal cortex. Aldosterone leads to an increase in blood sodium concentration, blood volume and therefore blood pressure. Once the blood pressure is regained, a negative feedback loop causes less renin to be secreted once more, and in this way the renin–angiotensin–aldosterone system contributes to fluid and electrolyte balance and blood pressure maintenance. In addition to stimulating aldosterone secretion, angiotensin II increases blood volume by stimulating thirst and therefore drinking. Angiotensin II also stimulates ADH release from the posterior pituitary gland and increases sodium ion reabsorption in the proximal convoluted tubules (Lote 1993).

Atrial natriuretic peptide

Atrial natriuretic peptide (ANP) also plays an important role in fluid and electrolyte balance. Natriuretic means 'sodium excreting', and ANP increases sodium ion loss from the body when appropriate by inhibiting sodium reabsorption in the kidney tubules (Jackson et al 2000). ANP is secreted from the atria of the heart in response to increased blood volume, which stretches the atria walls. ANP subsequently causes excretion of sodium ions and water to restore fluid volume and pressure. There are two other natriuretic peptides and all three of them have a range of effects on the heart, kidneys and central nervous system (Jackson et al 2000).

Consumption of salt in Western diets is about 10 g per day, and dietary salt seems to play a key role in hypertension. Mechanisms to excrete excess salt, including the role of ANP, may not be able to cope, leading to an increase in extracellular fluid and an increase in blood pressure. The increased blood pressure may then cause renal damage, which has a spiralling effect, increasing the blood pressure still further. A reduction in salt in the diet may not only reduce blood pressure in individuals with hypertension, but is also an important health promotion message for all (de Wardener 2000).

Hypersecretion and hyposecretion of hormones

There are many endocrine disorders, including those that result from too much (hypersecretion) or too little (hyposecretion) hormone secretion. Hyposecretion can be due to destruction of the endocrine gland tissue. This is often caused by autoimmune disease, in which immune responses are directed against the body's own tissues leading to their destruction. An example of endocrine dysfunction caused by autoimmunity is type 1 diabetes mellitus in which insulin-secreting cells of the pancreas are destroyed. Excessive hormone secretion can be caused by endocrine tumours, hyperplasia (excessive growth of cells) and autoimmune stimulation. For example, in Graves' disease (hyperthyroidism), excess thyroid hormone secretion results from autoantibodies (antibodies directed against 'self') being targeted at thyroid-specific proteins (Endo et al 1996). Some endocrine disorders are due to a change in hormone sensitivity by target cells rather than an increase or decrease in hormone secretion.

Hormone replacement therapy

Hormone replacement therapy (HRT), as the name suggests, replaces hormones. HRT is mainly associated with replacing hormones after the menopause, but other hormones, such as growth hormone and thyroid hormones, can also be 'replaced' in appropriate circumstances. Oestrogen and progesterone are secreted in much smaller amounts after the menopause and these are replaced to some extent by HRT (Bastin 1998). Appreciating the roles of oestrogen and progesterone in reproductive functions (see Ch. 9) will help you to understand the significance of replacing hormones following the menopause.

The menopause usually occurs somewhere between 48–56 years and results in the cessation of ovulation and menstruation. The climacteric is the transition time leading up to the menopause. The lower levels of oestrogen produced during and after the menopause are responsible for menopausal symptoms such as hot flushes experienced by some women. Lower levels of progesterone contribute to irregular vaginal bleeding. Psychological symptoms associated with the menopause are likely to be multifactorial, but the oestrogen deficiency does have a direct effect on the central nervous system.

The reduced levels of oestrogen after the menopause predispose women to osteoporosis (introduced in Ch. 2) and cardiovascular disease (Shaw 2001). The link between oestrogen deficiency and coronary heart disease is that the balance between HDL (high density lipoproteins) and low density lipoproteins (LDL) is upset (see p. 75). HDLs have a protective influence on the cardiovascular system (Libby 2002) and their levels decrease after the menopause (Bastin 1998).

HRT for postmenopausal women is a complex and contemporary topic. HRT can be either oestrogen alone or oestrogen plus progesterone (Burkman et al 2001). HRT enhances the profile of lipoproteins by reducing LDLs and increasing HDLs. HDLs are protective against the development of atherosclerosis and heart disease (Berra 2000). There are many other potential benefits of HRT including prevention of osteoporosis, reduced risk of colorectal cancer and Alzheimer's disease. These have to be balanced against the risks associated with HRT, the most important being an increased risk of breast cancer (Burkman et al 2001).

Sex hormones and cancer

Sex hormones are implicated in cancers of the breast, endometrium (lining of the uterus) and prostate (Tripathy & Benz 2001). Breast cancer is the most

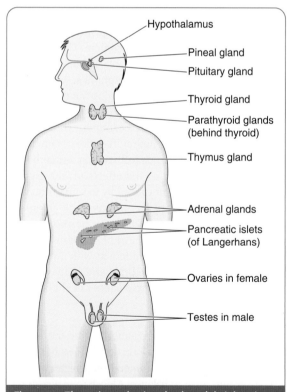

Figure 4.4 The major endocrine glands and their location in the body.

Reproduced with kind permission from Waugh & Grant 2001.

Table 4.1 Overview of endocrine glands and the key roles of hormones

Metabolic function	Hormones	Endocrine gland or tissue
Control of metabolic rate	Thyroxine (T_4) and tri-iodothyronine (T_3)	Thyroid gland
	Adrenaline and noradrenaline	Adrenal medulla
Control of calcium homeostasis	Parathyroid hormone	Parathyroid glands
	Calcitonin	Thyroid gland
	Active vitamin D	Kidneys and skin
Control of glucose homeostasis	Insulin and glucagon	Pancreatic islets
	Cortisol	Adrenal cortex
	Adrenaline and noradrenaline	Adrenal medulla
Fluid and electrolyte balance	Antidiuretic hormone	Posterior pituitary gland
	Aldosterone	Adrenal cortex
	Atrial natriuretic peptide	Atria
Responses to environment	Cortisol	Adrenal cortex
	Adrenaline and noradrenaline	Adrenal medulla
	Thymosin	Thymus
	Melatonin	Pineal gland
Growth and development	Growth hormone plus other trophic hormones	Anterior pituitary gland
	Thyroxine (T_4) and tri-iodothyronine (T_3)	Thyroid gland
	Oestrogen, progesterone and testosterone	Gonads
	Cortisol	Adrenal cortex
	Insulin	Pancreatic islets
	Active vitamin D	Skin and kidneys
Reproductive activities	Luteinizing hormone, follicle-stimulating hormone, prolactin	Anterior pituitary gland
	Oxytocin	Posterior pituitary gland
	Oestrogen, progesterone and testosterone	Gonads

common cancer in women (see p. 136) and oestrogen exposure is an important risk factor. This could be due to high levels of oestrogen or oestrogen peaks associated with a long period of reproductive life resulting from early menarche and late menopause (Debuse 1998). Oestrogen is a key stimulant in breast cancer interacting with target cells via nuclear oestrogen receptors. The presence of oestrogen receptors in breast cancer means the cancer may respond to hormonal therapy. Drugs such as tamoxifen that prevent oestrogen interacting with its nuclear receptors are called antioestrogens. Tamoxifen therapy is used in the management of oestrogen receptor positive cancers (Speirs and Kerin 2000).

To summarize, hormones are responsible for a diverse range of metabolic functions which are controlled in a coordinated way to maintain homeostasis and health. Hormones involved in homeostasis, stress, sleep and growth are discussed in other chapters in this book, demonstrating their crucial role in health. There are many other endocrine glands (see Fig. 4.4), tissues and hormones that have not been included in this chapter. A summary of hormones involved in a wide range of metabolic processes is given in Table 4.1.

Introducing the urinary system

The urinary system consists of the kidneys, which form urine and regulate fluid balance, the ureters, which transport urine to the bladder, a storage organ, and the urethra, which carries urine to the outside (see Fig. 4.5). The kidneys are reddish-brown bean-shaped organs found on the posterior wall of the abdominal cavity behind the peritoneum. The kidneys are encased in a protective layer of hard renal fat.

The kidneys are involved in excretion (removal of metabolic waste) and osmoregulation (regulation of the volume and composition of body fluids). The kidneys also contribute to homeostasis by secreting the hormone erythropoietin to control erythropoiesis (see Ch. 2). They also help to regulate pH and blood pressure, and activate vitamin D in calcium homeostasis (see Ch. 2).

The kidney has two distinct areas of tissue, the outer cortex and inner medulla (see Fig. 4.5). The medulla contains 8–18 wedge-shaped structures called medullary or renal pyramids. There is an internal funnel-shaped cavity called the renal pelvis which is divided into cup-like channels known as calyces.

Form and function of the nephron

The functional unit of the kidney is the nephron, composed of a kidney tubule and an associated blood capillary network (see Fig. 4.6). There are approximately one million nephrons in each kidney.

The structure of the tubules relate well to their function. Each tubule begins with a cup-shaped, Bowman's capsule, a double layer of squamous epithelium modified to act like a sieve. This connects to a coiled region, the proximal convoluted tubule, which has numerous microvilli, increasing the surface area of the lumen so that reabsorption of certain filtered substances can occur. The tubule then goes into a straight portion with a U-bend, called the loop of Henle. The tubule then becomes highly coiled again forming the distal convoluted tubule. Several distal convoluted tubules join to form a collecting duct and this gets progressively larger as more collecting ducts join it. The collecting ducts carry urine into the pelvis of the kidney.

The blood supply to each nephron consists of an afferent (incoming) arteriole that divides into a glomerulus, a knot of capillaries. These capillaries reunite to form an efferent (outgoing) arteriole. A capillary network leads off the efferent arteriole and lies close to the kidney tubule.

Urine formation in the nephron involves three processes. First, filtration of blood allowing certain substances into the tubule, next, reabsorption back into the blood of some of these filtered substances and finally, secretion of substances into the tubule from the surrounding blood capillaries.

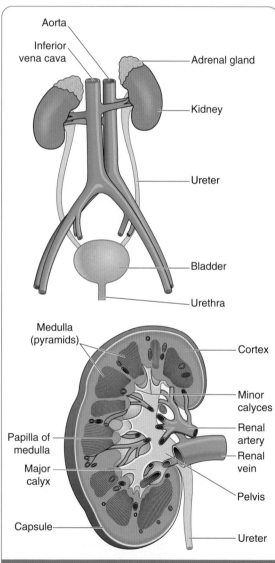

Figure 4.5 Urinary system.

The location of the organs of the urinary system is illustrated and the internal structure of the kidney is revealed. (Diagram of kidney reproduced with kind permission from Waugh & Grant 2001.)

Filtration

Blood is filtered by the filtration membrane, which consists of the glomerular capillary wall and the Bowman's

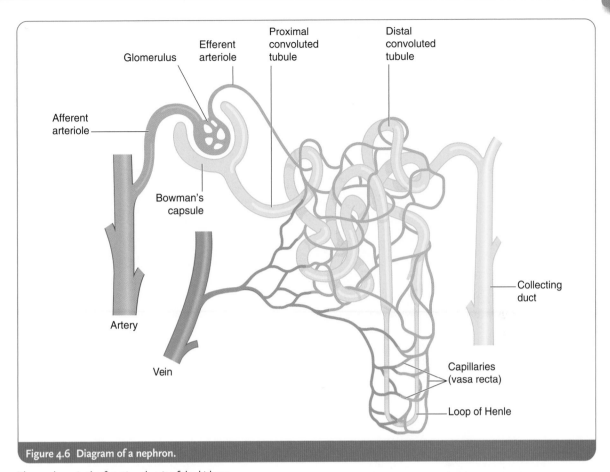

Figure 4.6 Diagram of a nephron.

The nephron is the functional unit of the kidney.

capsule. The glomerular capillary wall (endothelium) is modified to act as a filter; the presence of tiny pores, called fenestrae, make it more permeable than other capillaries. The basement membrane acts as a molecular sieve, filtering out large molecules and cells (Grant 2001). The epithelium of the Bowman's capsule contains modified epithelial cells called podocytes (see Fig. 4.7). These cells are shaped like octopi with several thick arms. Each arm has numerous little extensions called pedicels that wrap around the capillaries. This results in an epithelium with many gaps or slits that help to form the filter. The glomerular endothelium, basement membrane and podocytic epithelium of the Bowman's capsule form a selective filtration membrane that allows the passage of small molecules, but not the passage of large molecules, cells and cell fragments.

As illustrated in Figure 4.6, the afferent arteriole has a wider diameter than the efferent arteriole, which results in an increased pressure in the glomerular capillaries. This pressure tends to force water and small molecules out of blood into the Bowman's capsule

across the filtration membrane in a process called ultra-filtration. Glomerular filtrate contains water, glucose, amino acids, numerous ions and metabolites, including urea, uric acid, creatine and creatinine.

The rate of glomerular filtration is regulated by negative feedback mechanisms involving the juxta-glomerular apparatus. This comprises two cell types: renin-secreting cells located in the wall of the afferent arteriole, and the macula densa cells, which are special-ized muscle cells found in the epithelium of the distal convoluted tubule. On average the glomerular filtration rate (GFR) is about 125 ml min^{-1}, which corresponds to 180 litres in 24 hours (Lote 1993). It is important that the rate is maintained, otherwise toxic metabolic sub-stances such as urea, uric acid and creatinine would accumulate in the body. If the glomerular filtration rate falls the macula densa cells react by causing the afferent arteriole to dilate. This allows more blood to flow into the glomerulus and the GFR increases. At the same time the renin-secreting cells are stimulated to secrete renin. Renin is an enzyme that converts angiotensinogen, a

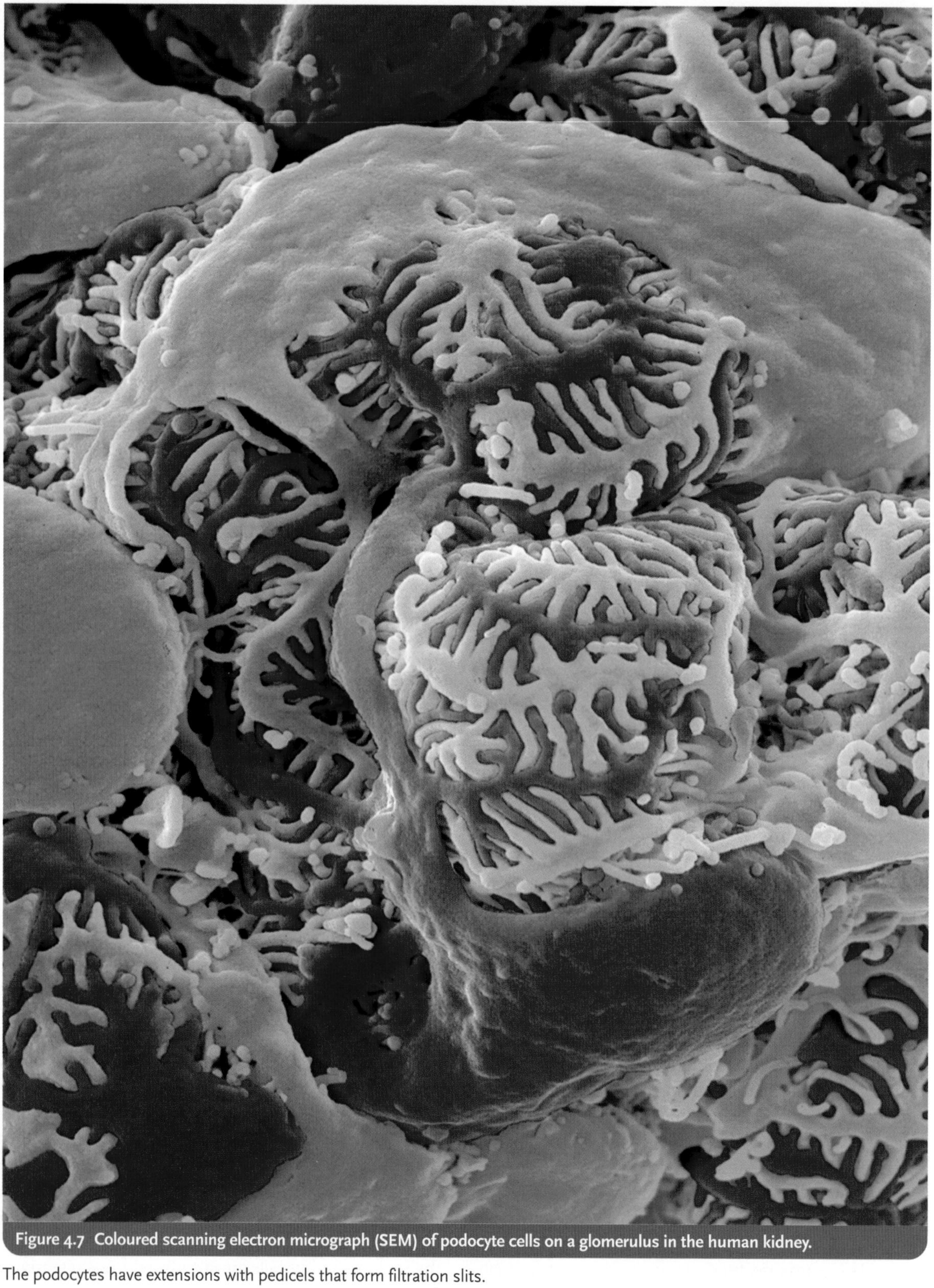

Figure 4.7 Coloured scanning electron micrograph (SEM) of podocyte cells on a glomerulus in the human kidney.

The podocytes have extensions with pedicels that form filtration slits.

plasma protein, into angiotensin I. Angiotensin I is then converted into angiotensin II, a potent vasoconstrictor, by a converting enzyme in the lungs (see Fig. 4.3). Angiotensin II causes vasoconstriction of the efferent arteriole, which leads to an increase in glomerular pressure and therefore GFR. In addition, angiotensin II has a number of other roles, including stimulating aldosterone release from the adrenal cortex and antidiuretic hormone release from the posterior pituitary gland. Both hormones play a key role in fluid balance.

The renin–angiotensin–aldosterone system is the main way in which the body responds to changes in blood volume and pressure (Beevers et al 2001, Lote 1993). Drugs that inhibit the action of angiotensin-converting enzyme are called ACE inhibitors and are effective in the treatment of heart failure. This is thought to be due to the combined effect of inhibition of angiotensin II (a vasoconstrictor) and an increase in bradykinin (a vasodilator). Angiotensin II also stimulates sympathetic activity of the cardiovascular system and ACE inhibitors will reduce this effect, with beneficial results (Davies et al 2000).

Reabsorption and secretion

Since small molecules such as glucose and amino acids are filtered out of blood along with urea and other metabolic waste, the nephron is adapted to reabsorb specific substances so that they are not lost from the body in urine. Most reabsorption occurs in the proximal convoluted tubule, a process enhanced by the numerous microvilli. Different parts of the tubule are adapted to reabsorb different substances by specific transport mechanisms. For example, most glucose is reabsorbed in the proximal convoluted tubule by active transport whilst most sodium ions are reabsorbed in the distal convoluted tubule by active transport. Reabsorption of sodium ions and water is controlled by a number of hormones discussed earlier in this chapter.

Active secretion of substances occurs from the capillary into the kidney tubule. Substances that may be secreted include hydrogen ions, potassium ions, ammonia, uric acid, creatinine and certain drugs.

The composition of urine is variable and depends on diet and level of activity. About 95% of urine is water, with a number of substances that result from metabolic reactions. These metabolic wastes include urea from the metabolism of amino acids in the liver, creatinine from the metabolism of creatine, and uric acid from the metabolism of nucleic acids. Urine also contains a range of electrolytes.

Urine formed by the nephrons collects in the pelvis of the kidney and flows by peristalsis along ureters to the bladder. The bladder can accommodate large amounts of urine until micturition (urination). It has a stretch lining of transitional epithelium and a muscular wall. There are two sphincters that control the flow of urine into the urethra: the internal sphincter is smooth muscle and the external sphincter is striped muscle under voluntary control. When the bladder contains about 400 ml of urine, stretch receptors initiate the micturition reflex.

References

Alescio-Lautier B, Paban V, Soumireu-Mourat B 2000 Neuromodulation of memory in the hippocampus by vasopressin. European Journal of Pharmacology 405(1–3):63–72

Asplund R, Aberg H 1991 Diurnal variation in the levels of antidiuretic hormone in the elderly. Journal of Internal Medicine 229(2):131–134

Bastin J 1998 Menopause – the end of fertility? Biological Sciences Review 11(2):15–18

Baxter J D, Ribeiro R C J 2001 Introduction to endocrinology. In: Greenspan F S, Gardner D G (eds) Basic and clinical endocrinology, 6th edn. Lange Medical/McGraw-Hill, New York, p 1–37

Beevers G, Lip G Y H, O'Brien E 2001 The pathophysiology of hypertension. British Medical Journal 322(7291):912–916

Berra K 2000 Women, coronary heart disease and dyslipidemia: does gender alter detection, evaluation or therapy? Journal of Cardiovascular Nursing 14(2):59–78

Burkman R T, Collins J A, Greene R A 2001 Current perspectives on benefits and risks of hormone replacement therapy. American Journal of Obstetrics and Gynecology 185(2): S13–S23

Davies M K, Gibbs C R, Lip G Y H 2000 Management: diuretics, ACE inhibitors, and nitrates. British Medical Journal 320(7232):428–431

Debuse M 1998 Endocrine and reproductive systems. Mosby International, London

de Wardener H 2000 Salt – the origin of hypertension. Biological Sciences Review 12(5):35–37

Endo T, Kogai T, Nakazato M et al 1996 Autoantibody against Na^+/I^- symporter in the sera of patients with autoimmune thyroid disease. Biochemistry and Biophysics Research Communications 224:92–95

Farrar E, Balment R 1990 Saving water! Biological Sciences Review 2(4):21–24

Fausto-Sterling A 1992 Myths of gender biological theories about women and men, 2nd edn. Basic Books, New York

Firestein S 2001 How the olfactory system makes sense of scents. Nature 413(6582):211–218

Funk C D 2001 Prostaglandins and leukotrienes: advances in eicosanoid biology. Science 294(5548):1871–1875

Gardner D G 2001 Mechanisms of hormone action. In: Greenspan F S, Gardner D G (eds). Basic and clinical endocrinology, 6th edn. Lange Medical/McGraw-Hill, New York, p 59–79

Grant M 2001 Basement membranes. Biological Sciences Review 13(4):36–39

Griffiths E 1993 The pituitary gland and homeostasis. Biological Sciences Review 5(3):25–27

Jackson G, Gibbs C R, Davies M K, Lip G Y H 2000 ABC of heart failure. Pathophysiology. British Medical Journal 320(7228): 167–170

Keverne E B 1999 The vomeronasal organ. Science 286(5440): 716–720

Kozono D, Masato Y, King L S, Agre P 2002 Aquaporin water channels: atomic structure and molecular dynamics meet clinical medicine. Journal of Clinical Investigation 109(11): 1395–1399

Libby P 2002 Atherosclerosis: the new view. Scientific American 286(5):30–37

Loffing J, Summa V, Zecevic M, Verrey F 2001 Mediators of aldosterone action in the renal tubule. Current Opinion in Nephrology and Hypertension 10(5):667–675

Lose G, Alling-Møller L, Jennum P 2001 Nocturia in women. American Journal of Obstetrics and Gynecology 185(2): 514–521

Lote C 1993 The kidney's balancing act. Biological Sciences Review 5(3):20–23

McCrone J 2000 Rebels without a cause. New Scientist 165(2222):22–27

McPherson H 2000 Tyrosine. Biological Sciences Review 12(4):29–30

Motluk A 2001 Scent of a man. New Scientist 169(2277):36–40

Shaw H 2001 Menopause. Biological Sciences Review 14(1):2–6

Sherman S I 2003 Thyroid carcinoma. Lancet 361:501–511

Small M F 1999 Nosing out a mate. Scientific American Presents 10(3):52–55

Steward M 1996 Water channels in the cell membrane. Biological Sciences Review 9(2):18–22

Speirs V, Kerin M J 2000 Prognostic significance of oestrogen receptor (beta) in breast cancer. British Journal of Surgery 87(4):405–409

Taylor R 1997 The sixth sense. New Scientist 153(2066):36–40

Townsend S 1982 The secret diary of Adrian Mole aged 13¼. Arrow, London, p 46

Tripathy D, Benz C C 2001 Hormones and cancer. In: Greenspan F S, Gardner D G (eds) Basic and clinical endocrinology, 6th edn. Lange Medical/McGraw-Hill, New York, p 762–777

Tsai M J, O'Malley B W 1994 Molecular mechanisms of action of steroid/thyroid receptor superfamily members. Annual Review of Biochemistry 63:451–486

Waugh A, Grant A 2001 Ross and Wilson: Anatomy and physiology in health and illness. Churchill Livingstone, Edinburgh

Weller A 1998 Human pheromones: communication through body odour. Nature 392(6672):126–127

Westwood M 1999 A receptor. Biological Sciences Review 12(2):6–7

Wiese J, Shlipak M G, Browner W S 2000 The alcohol hangover. Annals of Internal Medicine 132(11):897–902

5
NEUROTRANSMITTERS

❝The opportunities for subtle interactions between competing and collaborative nerve endings are thus almost unbelievably large. It is equally remarkable that any consistent behavioural pattern ever emerges from such a tangled mass of connections.❞

(Donovan 1988)

Coordination of cellular activities and integrated functioning of all organ systems is necessary to maintain homeostasis and a stable internal environment. This regulation of the internal environment is achieved by hormonal and neural mechanisms. Hormones, introduced in the previous chapter, are chemical messengers that control activity in target cells, whilst nerve fibres carry electrical impulses to effectors causing responses that maintain homeostasis. However, coordination by the nervous system is also achieved by chemicals since the majority of nerve cells elicit their responses by releasing chemicals called neurotransmitters onto receiving cells. There are many different types of neurotransmitter molecules, including acetylcholine, amines such as dopamine, amino acids of which glutamate is an important example, and a range of peptides including endorphins (Table 5.1) (Brotchie 1992).

Nerve cells, or neurons, play a key role in communication because they carry messages around the body and because groups of neurons in the brain are able to combine and integrate information from a range of sources. The scale of connections between neurons is hard to imagine – in the brain there are in the region of 10^{11} neurons and about 10^{14} connections or synapses in total (McCrohan 2001).

Some nerve cells in the brain make more than 20,000 connections with other nerve cells (Donovan 1988). Both ends of the neuron are adapted to enhance communication. The cell body of the neuron is covered in fine processes called dendrites that increase the surface area of the neuron so that it can receive information from many other neurons. The axon, a long process emerging from the cell body, is branched at its end forming the axon terminal, which because of its increased surface area is able to make many connections with other nerve cells, muscle cells or gland cells.

Structure and function of synapses

The connections between nerve cells are called synapses. Neurons communicate with each other by sending electrical impulses along their axons to the synapse, where chemical signals influence the dendrites and cell bodies of other neurons. The electrical signals, called action potentials, are unable to jump from one nerve cell to another; the information flows across the small space between the two adjacent nerve cells by the transfer of neurotransmitter molecules.

There are in fact two types of synapse, the type just described are called chemical synapses and are the most common. In electrical synapses the two nerve cells are very close together and connected by gap junctions through which the electrical signals can pass directly (McCrohan 2001).

Chemical synapses do not simply pass on the information, but play a crucial role in

Table 5.1 Classes of neurotransmitters				
Acetylcholine	Amines	Amino acids	Peptides	Gases
	Serotonin	Glutamate	Substance P	Nitric oxide
	Dopamine	Glycine	β Endorphin	
	Noradrenaline	GABA	Dynorphin	
	Adrenaline		Corticotrophin-releasing hormone (CRH)	

Note: There are several categories of neurotransmitters based on their chemical structure and a few examples are shown in their appropriate class. Acetylcholine is in a group by itself.

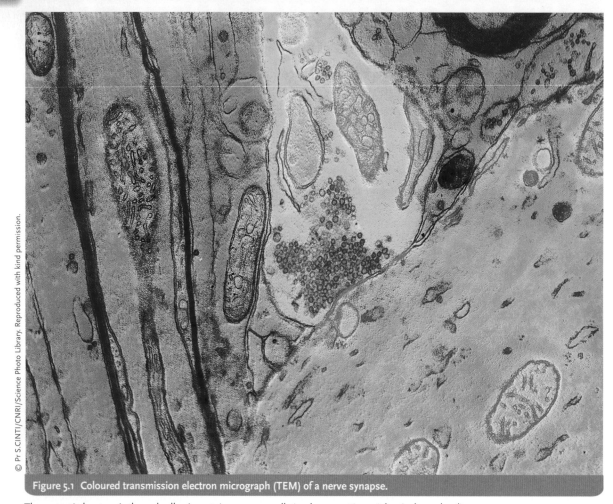

Figure 5.1 Coloured transmission electron micrograph (TEM) of a nerve synapse.

The synaptic bouton (coloured yellow) contains many small circular synaptic vesicles (coloured red).

processing information. Neurotransmitters travel from one neuron across a small gap (about 20–50 nm) and attach to receptors on the surface of the second neuron (Bendall 2003). This binding leads to intracellular changes that stimulate or inhibit firing of nerve impulses by the second neuron. Some transmitters produce rapid and short-term effects whilst others have effects that are slow in onset and longer in duration. Some neurotransmitters are excitatory and increase the likelihood of the receiving neuron sending messages onward, whilst others are inhibitory, making the second neuron less likely to fire off nerve impulses.

The axon terminal end branches have swollen tips called synaptic boutons. These contain synaptic vesicles, small membrane-bound sacs that contain the stored neurotransmitter molecules (see Fig. 5.1). Some neurotransmitters, the peptides, are synthesized in ribosomes in the cell body of the neuron and are transported along the axon to the terminal. Simpler neurotransmitters such as amino acids are made within the synaptic boutons.

Synaptic transmission

When a nerve impulse travelling along a presynaptic neuron reaches the axon terminal it triggers the opening of calcium channels in the membrane of that neuron. The influx of calcium ions causes the vesicles and their contents to move to the plasma membrane and fuse with it. This releases the neurotransmitter molecules into the synaptic gap or cleft (see Fig. 5.2). The neurotransmitter molecules diffuse across the space between the two neurons and bind with specific receptor proteins on the membrane of the postsynaptic neuron that of changes in the postsynaptic neuron including the opening of ion channels in the plasma membrane. These receptors enable more complex and long-lasting effects to occur in the postsynaptic neuron (Greengard 2001, McCrohan 2001).

Once the neurotransmitter has elicited a response in the postsynaptic neuron it is removed. Neurotransmitter molecules can be transported back in to the presynaptic terminal by transporter proteins in a process called re-uptake, or be inactivated by enzymes that break the large molecules into smaller inactivate fragments (Brotchie 1992).

Postsynaptic potentials

When neurotransmitters interact with receptors linked to ion channels on the postsynaptic membrane of the receiving neuron they produce postsynaptic potentials. These small electrical signals, approximately 1–2 mV, can vary in intensity and are short-lived, moving small distances across the cell membrane for a matter of one to several milliseconds. These postsynaptic potentials can be excitatory or inhibitory.

Excitatory postsynaptic potentials (EPSPs) are stimulated by excitatory neurotransmitters. As the neurotransmitter interacts with its receptor, sodium channels begin to open, causing a slight depolarization (reversal of electrical charges) that lowers the membrane potential, making the nerve cell more excitable. If enough EPSPs arrive more or less simultaneously an action potential will be generated in the postsynaptic neuron.

Inhibitory neurotransmitters have the opposite effect on the postsynaptic neuron making it less likely to fire off nerve impulses. Inhibitory neurotransmitters cause hyperpolarization of the postsynaptic membrane by eliciting the opening of chloride channels, allowing the negatively charged chloride ions to flow in, or by opening potassium channels, allowing positively charged potassium ions to leave. This makes the postsynaptic neuron much less responsive to excitatory potentials and less likely to fire action potentials (see Fig. 5.3).

Neurotransmitter molecules and their roles

There are many neurotransmitters, somewhere in the region of 50 to 100 representing different chemical types. As indicated earlier, most neurotransmitters are amines, peptides or amino acids (see Table 5.1). There is also a more novel group consisting of gases such as nitric oxide that are thought to be involved in

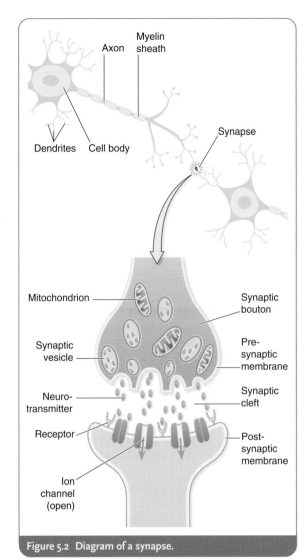

Figure 5.2 Diagram of a synapse.

On arrival of an action potential at the synaptic bouton, calcium ions flow in and trigger the synaptic vesicles to secrete their contents into the synaptic cleft. The neurotransmitter molecules bind to receptors on the postsynaptic membrane stimulating the opening of ion channels.

have the appropriate complementary shape. Once bound, the neurotransmitter causes the receptor to change shape. This change will eventually either excite or inhibit the postsynaptic neuron leading to an increase or decrease in the nerve impulses it generates.

There are two types of receptor on the postsynaptic membrane; one kind is directly linked to ion channels in the postsynaptic membrane whilst the other type of receptor signals the production of a second messenger (see p. 44). The second messenger can lead to a variety neurotransmission (Snyder & Ferris 2000). Noradrenaline, adrenaline and dopamine are sometimes collectively called the catecholamines.

Whilst the traditional model of neurons in the brain is that they make connections at synapses and use chemical transmitter substances to cross the gap, other mechanisms for communication have been proposed. For example, nerve cells may be able to communicate with other nerve cells by secreting chemicals directly into the extracellular space, the microenvironment of nerve cells in the brain, in a process known as volume transmission (Zoli et al 1998, Syková & Chvátal 2000).

Some of the evidence for communication between nerve cells at locations remote from synapses is the presence of receptors for neurotransmitters along the length of the axon, suggesting that chemicals could get there by volume transmission. In addition, some of the more novel neurotransmitters such as nitric oxide (which is a gas) probably use other signalling mechanisms, reinforcing the view that there may be other types of communication in the brain in addition to synaptic neurotransmission (Mitchell 1999).

> A smoke seemed to be going up from my nerves like the smoke from the grills and the sun-saturated road. The whole landscape – beach and headland and sea and rock – quavered in front of my eyes like a stage backcloth.
>
> (Sylvia Plath 1963)

Nevertheless, the crucial role of synapses and neurotransmission is not in doubt. Neurotransmitters are the key signalling molecules in the brain, they are hugely significant to health and many drugs exert their therapeutic actions by interfering with some aspect of neurotransmission. Dysfunctional synapses with altered secretion of neurotransmitters or a change in the number or sensitivity of receptors are implicated in a range of diseases, such as Parkinson's disease, Alzheimer's disease, depression and schizophrenia.

The most important excitatory neurotransmitter in the central nervous system is an amino acid, glutamate (Rorsman & Renström 1999). Glutamate contributes to learning and synaptic plasticity, a concept that will be discussed later. Neurons that use glutamate as their neurotransmitter are important excitatory pathways linking various parts of the brain, including the cortex, limbic system and thalamus. When glutamate binds to its receptors it enables sodium ions to flow into the postsynaptic neuron, causing depolarization and an excitatory signal to be generated. There are two major types of glutamate receptor, the AMPA (amino-3-hydroxy-5-methyl-4-isoxazole propionate) receptor and the NMDA (N-methyl-D-aspartate) receptor. The AMPA receptor incorporates an ion channel that opens following glutamate binding. AMPA receptors have an important role in determining the strength of synaptic transmission in the

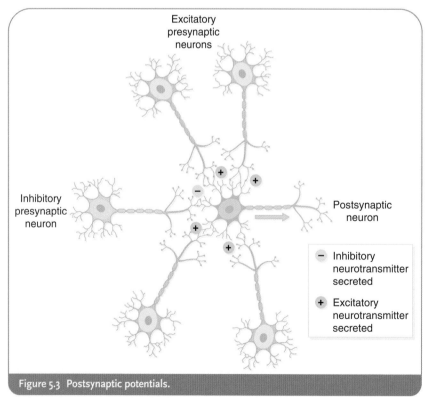

Excitatory presynaptic neurons

Inhibitory presynaptic neuron

Postsynaptic neuron

− Inhibitory neurotransmitter secreted

+ Excitatory neurotransmitter secreted

Figure 5.3 Postsynaptic potentials.

In this illustration, the postsynaptic neuron is receiving both inhibitory and excitatory inputs at the same time. The individual postsynaptic potentials are added together. The excitatory postsynaptic potentials predominate and so the postsynaptic neuron is excited and action potentials are generated.

brain and can wander around on the surface of neurons. When AMPA receptors accumulate at synapses they increase postsynaptic excitation and when they are removed they depress or inhibit synaptic neurotransmission (Sheng & Nakagawa 2002). NMDA receptors are involved in memory (Bendall 2003).

The activity of glutamate in synapses depends on the balance between glutamate reuptake into the presynaptic neuron and receptor inactivation. Glutamate levels in synapses are regulated by glutamate transporters. Disturbed functioning of glutamate transporters is implicated in Alzheimer's disease, brain cell death in cerebral ischaemia, and epilepsy (Maragakis & Rothstein 2001). NMDA receptors may also be involved in the pathophysiology of schizophrenia (Goff & Coyle 2001).

Not only is glutamate a neurotransmitter, but it also acts as an intracellular signal involved in insulin secretion from pancreatic β cells in response to glucose stimulation (Rorsman & Renström 1999). This emphasizes the multiplicity of roles that chemical signals have. In addition, some people seem to have a reaction following ingestion of glutamate in the form of monosodium glutamate, a flavour enhancer. The mechanism by which this ingested glutamate stimulates these effects is unknown but again reinforces the view that chemical signals have diverse roles. Symptoms include headache, flushing, numbness and tingling (Yang et al 1997).

GABA or gamma amino butyric acid is synthesized from glutamate in GABA-secreting neurons. GABA is secreted by many nerve endings in the brain; about 40% of synapses in the brain use GABA as the neurotransmitter. When GABA binds to its receptors it increases the opening of chloride channels. As more negatively charged chloride ions enter the postsynaptic neuron it becomes less excitable, which is why GABA is a powerful inhibitory neurotransmitter. GABA-secreting neurons are involved in sleep, muscle relaxation, anxiety reduction, and in the relaxing effects of alcohol (Hedaya 1996).

GABA seems to be an important neurotransmitter implicated in anxiety. Drugs used to treat anxiety, such as the benzodiazepines, target GABA receptors. Many neurotransmitters, including GABA, have a number of specific receptor sub-types. Benzodiazepines interact with $GABA_A$–benzodiazepine receptors. When benzodiazepines specifically target these receptors in certain areas of the brain, anxiety is reduced. The therapeutic effect of benzodiazepines results from them interacting with these GABA receptors and enhancing GABA effects. The postsynaptic neurons are inhibited and anxiety is reduced (Nutt & Malizia 2001).

Synaptic integration

The nervous system is responsible for filtering and integrating information; this is possible because of synapses. As emphasized earlier, synapses do not just pass on information, but integrate the information coming from a number of sources along different neurons. Nerve cells in the brain may be influenced via synapses with thousands of other brain cells. Some of the synapses will be excitatory and some will be inhibitory. Each neuron may receive hundreds of excitatory postsynaptic potentials and inhibitory postsynaptic potentials. In a process called summation, all the positive and negative inputs are added together to determine whether the postsynaptic neuron will send a signal or not. If the number of excitatory inputs overall are sufficiently great, it will transmit nerve impulses (McCrohan 2001) (see Fig. 5.3).

Synapses can enhance or reduce the strength of the signal; in most synapses the signal is dampened rather than amplified. Another aspect of synaptic integration is the ability of some synapses to change a short presynaptic signal into a prolonged postsynaptic signal. This often occurs when receptor binding leads to the generation of a second messenger in the postsynaptic neuron. This intracellular signal can have long-lasting effects (McCrohan 1996).

Synaptic plasticity

A most important characteristic of synapses is that they possess the ability to change their strength. This mechanism is thought to be the basis of learning and memory (McCrohan 1996). When information repeatedly flows along a neuronal circuit during a repetitive task, for example, the strength of the connections between the neurons involved increases and results in long-term changes in synaptic strength. There are three mechanisms that may contribute to this increase in synaptic strength: They are a change in:

- the amount of neurotransmitter released by the presynaptic neuron;
- the sensitivity of the postsynaptic membrane;
- the actual number of synapses between the presynaptic and postsynaptic neurons (McCrohan 1996).

Repetitive stimulation of some synapses in the brain increases the effectiveness of transmission at those synapses. When synapses in the brain increase their strength it is called long-term potentiation (LTP).

The mechanism has been studied extensively in the hippocampus. The hippocampus is a region in the brain involved in memory, reasoning, language and other cognitive functions. LTP results from a mechanism involving glutamate and NMDA receptors on the postsynaptic neuron (LeDoux 2002). Glutamate interacting with AMPA receptors on the postsynaptic membrane leads to NMDA receptor channels allowing calcium ions to flow in; the increase in calcium ion concentration is the critical trigger for LTP (Malenka & Nicoll 1999). For LTP to continue, gene expression and protein synthesis have to occur. Once LTP has occurred, nerve impulses travel more easily along the pathway. This describes the cellular mechanism on which learning and memory are based (Bendall 2003).

Plasticity in the developing brain

Plasticity suggests that the brain may be moulded or changed. Physical changes such as the number and extent of connections between neurons in the brain are changed by experiences (Kolb & Whishaw 1998, Greenfield 2000). Plasticity is very important in the developing brain. The number of neurons and synapses present in the fetal brain are in excess of those required later in life. Extraneous neurons and unused synapses are lost and the neuronal circuitry evolves in the first few years of life as the brain develops in response to stimulation from the external environment (Johnston et al 2001). As an illustration of how important our formative experiences are in shaping the developing brain, stress during childhood can lead to long-term changes, including mental illness. Childhood abuse elicits an array of hormonal effects that can modify brain development and the architecture of the brain. For example, exposure to stress hormones can change the number and shape of neurons in the hippocampus with long-term consequences (Teicher 2002).

The roles of a number of neurotransmitters will now be introduced, illustrating their diverse roles in health and disease. Acetylcholine, one of the first neurotransmitters to be studied, is implicated in memory and learning and a range of other behaviours including aggression, thirst and sexuality (Donovan 1988). Neurons that secrete acetylcholine at their synapse are called cholinergic neurons and are implicated in Alzheimer's disease (Gooch & Stennett 1996). Acetylcholine is the neurotransmitter involved in neuromuscular transmission explored later in this chapter. Myasthenia gravis is a disease in which this neuromuscular transmission is impaired because of the loss of functional acetylcholine receptors (Wittbrodt 1997).

Acetylcholine and Alzheimer's disease

It is estimated that by 2025, 22 million people in the world will have Alzheimer's disease (St. George-Hyslop 2000). This is the most common cause of dementia, occurring more frequently as people get older, and so as life expectancy increases more people are likely to have this condition. There are a number of changes in nerve cell structure and function that have been identified. Changes in the brain include the appearance of neuritic plaques and neurofibrillary tangles (see Ch. 1) together with the loss of cholinergic neurons in certain areas of the brain (Gooch & Stennett 1996). In Alzheimer's disease, the cholinergic neurons that project to the cortex and hippocampus from the basal forebrain die.

Cholinergic neurons secrete acetylcholine into the synaptic gap. Acetylcholine is rapidly broken down by an enzyme, acetylcholinesterase, into smaller inactive metabolites (Brotchie 1992). Drugs that block this enzyme, such as donepezil, rivastigmine and galantamine, help to conserve acetylcholine in the synapses and lead to some improvement in cognitive function in mild to moderate Alzheimer's disease (Bullock 2002). Other drugs are under development to manage the symptoms of Alzheimer's disease, including anti-inflammatory drugs, oestrogen and vitamin E (Bullock 2002) and NMDA antagonists for moderately severe to severe Alzheimer's disease (Kilpatrick & Tilbrook 2002). Many questions remain about the disease process and the efficacy of the treatments (Motluk 2003).

Serotonin and depression

Serotonin-producing neurons extend into many areas of the brain and have various roles, including the modulation of mood. Serotonin was so named because it was first isolated from blood serum and found to increase muscle tone in blood vessel walls. Serotonin or 5-hydroxytryptamine (5-HT), its chemical name, is synthesized in synaptic boutons from tryptophan, an amino acid that is essential in our diet (Kennett 1999). Tryptophan in its purified form has an antidepressant effect in mild-to-moderate depression although foods rich in tryptophan are not thought to raise brain tryptophan levels (Young 2002). Acute tryptophan depletion resulting from lack of tryptophan in the diet is associated with a fall in tryptophan levels in the brain, decreased serotonin synthesis and a lowering of mood, emphasizing the role of serotonin in mood regulation (Young 2002).

Once serotonin is synthesized, it is stored in synaptic vesicles and secreted into the synaptic cleft following arrival of nerve impulses in the synaptic bouton.

Serotonin binds to specific receptors on the post-synaptic membrane and influences the firing rate of the neuron. Serotonin is removed from the synaptic cleft by reuptake mechanisms so it can be reused or broken down into inactive metabolites by the enzyme monoamine oxidase. Drugs that inhibit this enzyme are called monoamine oxidase inhibitors (MAOIs) and are prescribed as antidepressants; they allow serotonin to accumulate in the synapse. Drugs such as fluoxetine (Prozac®) achieve a similar effect by blocking the reuptake of serotonin into the presynaptic neuron. They are called selective serotonin reuptake inhibitors (SSRIs) (Kennett 1999, Richelson 2001).

Parkinson's disease

Parkinson's disease is, after Alzheimer's disease, the commonest neurodegenerative disease with an estimated incidence of 20 in 100,000 (Schapira 1999). The disease is particularly characterized by tremor, rigidity and slowness of movements; these three features are attributed to disturbed muscle control. Loss of neurons in an area of the brain called the substantia nigra are implicated in the disease. Neurons in this region of the brain use dopamine as the neurotransmitter. Death of these dopaminergic neurons leads to a dopamine deficiency in the striatum (Barker et al 1998). The striatum forms part of the basal ganglia, a collection of structures found deep in the forebrain that exert control over muscle movements. Drugs used to treat the symptoms of Parkinson's disease are aimed at raising dopamine levels in the striatum. Levodopa is the most commonly used treatment for Parkinson's disease. This drug is able to cross the blood–brain barrier and once inside brain cells is converted into dopamine. Various other drugs may be used, including dopamine agonists, which mimic the actions of dopamine (Brooks 2000).

Neuromuscular junction

Motor neurons carry nerve impulses from the central nervous system to skeletal muscles; this means the axon terminal connects with a muscle cell rather than a nerve cell. The junction formed between a motor neuron and muscle cell is called a neuromuscular junction (see Fig. 5.4). The structure and functions of neuromuscular junctions are similar to synapses. The neurotransmitter molecule used in these neuromuscular junctions is

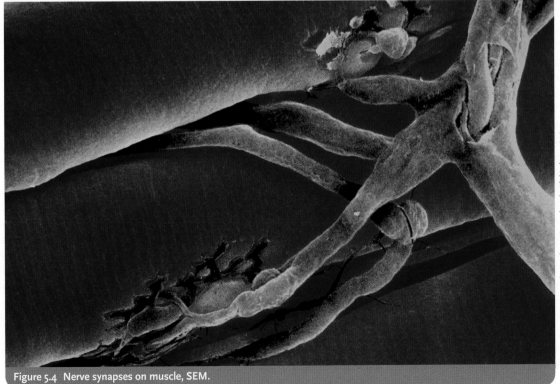

© Don Fawcett/Science Photo Library. Reproduced with kind permission.

Figure 5.4 Nerve synapses on muscle, SEM.

The motor neuron (green) ends in a group of pads called end plates. When activated, the end plates release the neurotransmitter acetylcholine, which makes the muscle fibres (red) contract.

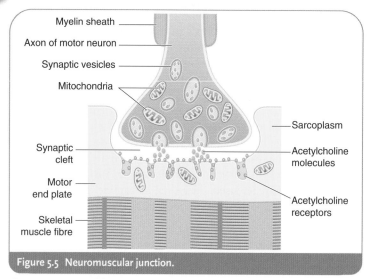

Figure 5.5 Neuromuscular junction.

The axon terminal of the motor neuron forms a synapse with a skeletal muscle fibre. Acetylcholine secreted from the presynaptic neuron stimulates receptors in the motor end plate.

the effects of ageing does seem paradoxical since it is a potent neurotoxin (Misra 2002).

Myasthenia gravis

Myasthenia gravis is a disorder of the neuromuscular junction in which transmission is impaired by the dysfunction of the acetylcholine receptors. The pathological mechanisms involved include autoimmunity in which the body's own immune system produces antibodies that disable the acetylcholine receptors so that neurotransmission is disturbed. The characteristic feature of myasthenia gravis caused by this impaired neurotransmission is skeletal muscle weakness, particularly during periods of activity. A range of drugs are used to improve neuromuscular transmission and increase muscle strength, these include cholinesterase inhibitors. These drugs block the action of acetylcholinesterase and thus allow acetylcholine to accumulate, enhancing neuromuscular transmission (Pruitt & Swift 2002).

acetylcholine, which when released from the axon terminal by the arrival of nerve impulses causes the muscle cell to contract.

Acetylcholine is synthesized in the synaptic boutons from choline and acetate under the influence of an enzyme, choline acetyl transferase. Adenosine triphosphate (ATP) from the numerous mitochondria in the presynaptic neuron supplies the necessary energy. The plasma membrane of the muscle cell or fibre is called the sarcolemma and this is folded extensively in the motor end plate (see Fig. 5.5).

Once acetylcholine is secreted into the synaptic cleft it interacts with specific receptors on the sarcolemma. This leads to the opening of sodium channels and depolarization, and in turn this activates the contractile proteins in the muscle fibre. The enzyme acetylcholinesterase located on both the neural membrane and the sarcolemma rapidly inactivates acetylcholine, forming acetate and choline, which are reabsorbed and recycled in the synaptic bouton.

Some people attempt to temporarily reduce wrinkles and animation lines in the face by disrupting neurotransmission in particular facial muscle fibres. Botulinum toxin type A (Botox) injections temporarily block acetylcholine secretion from the presynaptic neuron. This lack of neurotransmitter causes the muscle fibres to be effectively weakened or paralysed for a period of time. Animation lines can be reduced for about six months following treatment (Ellis et al 1997). Botulinum toxin does have therapeutic uses, but its popularity in masking

Introducing skeletal muscles

A skeletal muscle is an organ composed of bundles of elongated muscle cells, also known as fibres, which are bound together in bundles by connective tissue. Small blood vessels and nerve branches run through the connective tissue surrounding each muscle fibre. The whole muscle is also encased in connective tissue, which extends to form tendons that attach the muscle to bones.

The structure of skeletal muscle is based on long cylindrical structures that enclose progressively smaller cylindrical elements. A useful analogy is a set of wooden Russian dolls of increasingly smaller size which are made to fit inside one another. Each muscle fibre contains long cylindrical fibres called myofibrils and each myofibril contains two types of myofilaments, thick myosin and thin actin filaments (see Fig. 5.6).

Myofibrils have a banded appearance, which is why skeletal muscle is called 'striped' muscle. Thick and thin filaments overlap each other in alternate layers, creating bands, which form contractile units called sarcomeres. The thick myosin filaments have 'heads' mounted on long arms. Actin filaments have binding sites for these

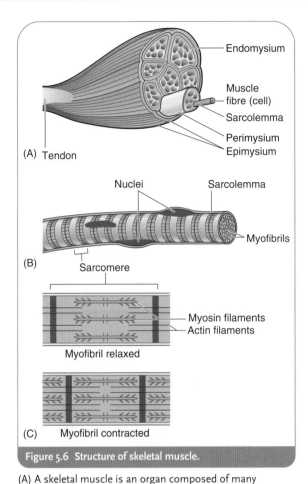

(A) Tendon

(B) Sarcomere

Myosin filaments
Actin filaments

Myofibril relaxed

(C) Myofibril contracted

Figure 5.6 Structure of skeletal muscle.

(A) A skeletal muscle is an organ composed of many bundles of muscle fibres enclosed in connective tissue.
(B) Each muscle fibre consists of smaller myofibrils.
(C) Myofibrils contain thick myosin and thin actin filaments.
(Reproduced with kind permission from Waugh & Grant 2001.)

myosin 'heads', but when the muscle is resting these sites are covered up by tropomyosin, which winds around the actin filament. Another protein, troponin, is attached to the tropomyosin at intervals.

Sliding filament model

A muscle contracts when the contractile units, sarcomeres, shorten. This occurs when the thick and thin filaments slide over one another. The filaments can slide over each other because the myosin heads form cross-bridges to actin filaments at the binding sites. The heads then rotate so that actin filaments are pulled towards the centre of the sarcomere and the filaments slide over each other and the sarcomeres shorten. The myosin head then detaches and reattaches at the next actin binding site; this process requires ATP and results in actin on each side of the sarcomere being brought closer together (Mills 1998).

The energy for these activities comes from ATP produced in the numerous mitochondria found in muscle cells. ATP binds to the cross-bridges between myosin heads and actin filaments. ATP enables the myosin heads to swivel and flip from one actin binding site to another. Because muscles cannot store much ATP they recycle the adenosine diphosphate (ADP) into ATP rapidly. Creatine phosphate is a muscle storage product that is involved in the rapid regeneration of ADP into ATP.

Calcium ions (Ca^{2+}) are required for muscle fibres to contract since myosin–actin interaction depends on their presence. When a muscle is stimulated to contract, Ca^{2+} is released into the sarcomere enabling the actin binding sites to become exposed. Ca^{2+} binds to troponin causing it to change shape and this in turn displaces tropomyosin leaving the actin binding sites free for myosin heads to bind. The entry of Ca^{2+} into the sarcoplasm and removal by pumps is therefore crucial in muscle contraction (Fry 1996).

Neuromuscular transmission leads to muscle fibre contraction

The action potential induces a sequence of events that leads to muscle contraction, this sequence is called excitation–contraction coupling. Nerve impulses are transmitted across the neuromuscular junction by acetylcholine resulting in a muscle action potential that travels deep into the muscle fibre via transverse tubules. The action potential causes Ca^{2+} to be released from sarcoplasmic reticulum. Ca^{2+} binds to troponin, which alters shape and moves the tropomyosin molecules uncovering the binding sites, linkages form between actin and myosin, and the muscle fibre shortens and contraction occurs. Relaxation occurs when calcium ions dissociate from troponin and are pumped back into the sarcoplasmic reticulum; this allows tropomyosin to resume its position, blocking the binding sites on the actin molecules. The muscle fibres then elongate by passive stretching.

All the individual muscle fibres contribute to skeletal muscle contraction; the strength of the contraction depends on how many individual muscle fibres contract and how frequently each muscle fibre is stimulated to contract (Fry 1996).

Muscle fibre types

There are many different types of fibre found in skeletal muscle (Bottinelli & Reggiani 2000). Despite the diversity, however, two main types of skeletal muscle fibre can be considered, the red slow-twitch fibres and white fast-twitch fibres, with their different colours reflecting differences in their metabolism. A twitch is a brief contraction of a muscle fibre in response to a single stimulus. Fast-twitch fibres respond quickly to stimulation and gain their energy by the glycolysis of intramuscular glycogen stores. They are pale because there is little myoglobin, a red pigment similar to haemoglobin that stores oxygen. Lactic acid builds up during contraction and results in muscle fatigue. Slow-twitch fibres get their energy from aerobic respiration; ATP is produced in the numerous mitochondria as a result of Krebs cycle and oxidative phosphorylation (Fry 1996). Because slow fibres use aerobic respiration they are fatigue resistant. Most skeletal muscles are a mixture of red and white fibres, because they carry out a range of functions. The slow fatigue-resistant red fibres are important for most slow and repeated activities and for maintaining posture, whilst fast white fibres are essential for short bursts of activity (Bottinelli & Reggiani 2000). The balance of these different muscle fibres is roughly equal in most people, but athletes who excel in endurance events tend to have a higher proportion of slow red fibres, whilst athletes who perform in short and very fast sports like sprinting or jumping have a preponderance of fast white fibres (Jones 1990).

> **When the time came both started off together, but the Hare was soon so far ahead that he thought he might as well have a rest: so down he lay and fell asleep. Meanwhile the Tortoise kept plodding on, and in time reached the goal. At last the Hare woke up with a start, and dashed on at his fastest, but only to find that the Tortoise had already won the race.**
>
> **Slow and steady wins the race.**
>
> ('The Hare and the Tortoise', Aesop)

Control of movement

Muscle movements are complicated, interdependent and coordinated. Muscles around a joint do not work in isolation; they often work together as a group. Muscles that initiate a particular movement are called prime movers and those that resist or counter their action are called antagonists. Synergists are muscles that stabilize the joint and assist the prime mover. The mechanisms involved in enabling us to make smooth, controlled and coordinated movements are complex and depend on the brain integrating lots of information. The brain is responsible for selecting the right combination of muscle movements; this is called the motor programme. The selection of the appropriate motor programme depends on information from a range of sources, including information about joint position and muscle tone. The next step is to initiate the motor programme and send out instructions via motor neurons to the skeletal muscle fibres. Once the movement has begun, adjustments are made based on continual feedback so that movement is controlled and coordinated throughout (Brotchie 2000).

Many areas of the brain contribute to the control of movement, including the basal ganglia which select and initiate the muscle programme, the motor cortex which sends signals to the muscles, and the cerebellum which coordinates the ongoing movements (Brotchie 2000). Any dysfunction in these areas causes movement disorders. In Parkinson's disease, for example, the disordered movement results from a problem in selecting the appropriate movement. This is due to the loss of dopamine-secreting neurons, which project from the substantia nigra to the basal ganglia as described earlier (Barker et al 1998).

In summary, nerve cells communicate with each other by synaptic transmission. There are a variety of excitatory and inhibitory neurotransmitters, which with their specific receptors are responsible for the integration and processing of information in the brain. Neurotransmitter molecules often have multiple roles. Neuromuscular junctions, where nerve fibres meet muscle fibres, function in a similar way. Acetylcholine is the neurotransmitter substance involved in signalling skeletal muscle fibres to contract. Dysfunctional synapses and neuromuscular junctions contribute to a range of diseases and many drugs exert their actions at these sites.

References

Aesop 1979 Aesop's Fables. Heinemann, London, p 92,95

Barker S, Grant A, Hodnicki D R 1998 Parkinson's disease: a holistic approach. American Journal of Nursing 98(11): 48A–48H

Bendall K 2003 This is your life.... New Scientist 178(2395): Inside Science 160

Bottinelli R, Reggiani C 2000 Human skeletal muscle fibres: molecular and functional diversity. Progress in Biophysics and Molecular Biology 73(2–4):195–262

Brooks D J 2000 Dopamine agonists: their role in the treatment of Parkinson's disease. Journal of Neurology, Neurosurgery and Psychiatry 68(6):685–689

Brotchie J 1992 Bridging the gap. Biological Sciences Review 5(1):35–39

Brotchie J 2000 Make a move. Biological Sciences Review 12(5):28–32

Bullock R 2002 New drugs for Alzheimer's disease and other dementias. British Journal of Psychiatry 180:135–139

Donovan B T 1988 Humors, hormones and the mind. Macmillan Press, London, p 42–43

Ellis D A, Chi P L, Tan A K W 1997 Facial rejuvenation with botulinum. Dermatology Nursing 9(5):329–333

Fry C 1996 The physiology of muscle. Biological Sciences Review 8(3):2–6

Goff D C, Coyle J T 2001 The emerging role of glutamate in the pathophysiology and treatment of schizophrenia. American Journal of Psychiatry 158(9):1367–1377

Gooch M D, Stennett D J 1996 Molecular basis of Alzheimer's disease. American Journal of Health-System Pharmacy 53(13):1545–1557

Greengard P 2001 The neurobiology of slow synaptic transmission. Science 294(5544):1024–1030

Greenfield S 2000 The private life of the brain. Penguin, London

Hedaya R J 1996 Understanding biological psychiatry. Norton, New York

Johnston M V, Nishimura A, Harum K et al 2001 Sculpting the developing brain. Advances in Pediatrics 48:1–38

Jones D 1990 The fast whites and the slower reds. Biological Sciences Review 2(4):2–6

Kennett G 1999 Serotonin – the brain's mood modulator. Biological Sciences Review 12(1):28–31

Kilpatrick G J, Tilbrook G S 2002 Memantine. Merz. Current Opinion in Investigational Drugs 3(5):798–806

Kolb B, Whishaw I Q 1998 Brain plasticity and behaviour. Annual Review of Psychology 49:43–64

LeDoux J E 2002 Emotion, memory and the brain. Scientific American 12(1):62–71

Malenka R C, Nicoll R A 1999 Long-term potentiation – a decade of progress? Science 285(5435):1870–1874

Maragakis N J, Rothstein J D 2001 Glutamate transporters in neurologic disease. Archives of Neurology 58(3):365–370

McCrohan C 1996 Synapses. Biological Sciences Review 8(4):26–29

McCrohan C 2001 Making the connection. Biological Sciences Review 13(3):10–13

Mills J 1998 Skeletal muscle – is bigger always better? Biological Sciences Review 11(2):36–39

Misra V P 2002 The changed image of botulinum toxin: its unlicensed use is increasing dramatically, ahead of robust evidence. British Medical Journal 325(7374):1188

Mitchell A 1999 Liquid genius. New Scientist 161(2177):26–30

Motluk A 2003 Fragile minds. New Scientist 177(2380):34–37

Nutt D J, Malizia A L 2001 New insights into the role of the $GABA_A$ – benzodiazepine receptor in psychiatric disorder. British Journal of Psychiatry 179:390–396

Plath S 1963 The bell jar. Faber & Faber, London, p 166

Pruitt J N, Swift T R 2002 Therapies for disorders of the neuromuscular junction. Archives of Neurology 59(5): 739–742

Rorsman P, Renström E 1999 Cell biology: glutamate primes the pump. Nature 402(6762):595–596

Richelson E 2001 Pharmacology of antidepressants. Mayo Clinic Proceedings 76(5):511–527

Schapira A H 1999 Science, medicine and the future: Parkinson's disease. British Medical Journal 18:311–314

Sheng M, Nakagawa T 2002 Neurobiology: glutamate receptors on the move. Nature 417(6889):601–602

Snyder S H, Ferris C D 2000 Novel neurotransmitters and their neuropyschiatric relevance. American Journal of Pyschiatry 157(11):1738–1751

St. George-Hyslop P H 2000 Piecing together Alzheimer's. Scientific American 283(6):52–59

Syková E, Chvátal A. Glial cells and volume transmission in the CNS. Neurochemistry International 36(4–5):397–409

Teicher M H 2002 Scars that won't heal: the neurobiology of child abuse. Scientific American 286(3):68–75

Waugh A, Grant A 2001 Ross and Wilson: Anatomy and physiology in health and illness. Churchill Livingstone, Edinburgh

Wittbrodt E T 1997 Drugs and myasthenia gravis. Archives of Internal Medicine 157(4):339–408

Yang W H, Drouin M, Herbert M et al 1997 The monosodium glutamate symptom complex: assessment in a double-blind, placebo-controlled, randomised study. Journal of Allergy and Clinical Immunology 99(6 Part 1):757–762

Young S N 2002 Clinical nutrition 3. The fuzzy boundary between nutrition and psychopharmacology. Canadian Medical Associan Journal 166(2):205–209

Zoli M, Torri C, Ferrari R et al 1998 The emergence of the volume transmission concept. Brain Research. Brain Research Reviews 26(2–3):136–147

6

STRESS

Stress is an inevitable facet of life. Stress is not necessarily harmful; indeed without a certain amount of stress it would be difficult to function. Although stress is a risk factor for a number of different diseases, good stresses promote health and wellbeing. Many theories and models have been developed to explain stress and its impacts on health (Rice 1992). In the response-based model of stress the emphasis is on the physiological and psychological responses to stressors. Stress is the body's response to a real or perceived threat. Stress refers to any demand that outstrips the individual's ability to cope. On the other hand, the notion of the individual's perception of threat being crucial to the stress response is central to the transactional model of stress (Lazarus & Folkman 1984). In this model, the person experiences stress when there is an imbalance between the perceived demands and the ability to cope with them. A stressor is a stress-producing factor or situation. Stressors are not necessarily physical, since psychological arousal such as fear and social factors such as poverty can also elicit the stress response.

Stress is a threat to homeostasis and being able to adapt to stress ensures survival. As discussed in Chapter 2, homeostasis is the maintenance of a dynamic equilibrium with the environment and involves physiological and behavioural responses. The stress response enables the individual to meet the perceived danger and involves virtually every organ system responding in an integrated fashion. All the changes that occur in response to a stressor are designed to promote homeostasis.

The response to stressors involves both the nervous and endocrine systems coordinating activities that counter stress. The brain recognizes and evaluates the danger and if appropriate activates the stress response system. This response involves an array of chemical signals including both hormones and neurotransmitters. These signals induce behavioural changes and mobilize energy that is directed towards the brain, muscles and stressed body sites; steps necessary to promote homeostasis (O'Connor et al 2000). In addition to hormones and neurotransmitters, other chemical signals called cytokines are also important in the stress response. Immune cells secrete cytokines in response to stressors

and these cytokines stimulate further production of stress hormones from the hypothalamus, anterior pituitary and adrenal cortex (Tsigos & Chrousos 2002, Yang & Glaser 2002).

There are two main thrusts to the neuroendocrine response to stressors. The rapid reaction to an immediate threat is often called the 'fight or flight' response and results from the effects of adrenaline secretion from the adrenal medulla and noradrenaline secretion from sympathetic nerve fibres, both of which prepare the body for physical exertion. This alarm reaction evolved in our ancestors to enable them to survive in hostile environments by fleeing or fighting a predator. In contemporary times the stressors can be physical, emotional, social and psychological. The alarm reaction occurs in modern humans to make us more alert and to prime the body for action (Cooper 1992, Brunner 1997). The other axis of the stress response system results in the secretion of cortisol from the adrenal cortex. Cortisol is involved in increasing metabolism and marshalling many components in the body including the cardiovascular, respiratory and immune systems to deal with the threat.

General adaptation syndrome

In the 1950s, Selye described the general adaptation syndrome, in which the response to stress is characterized by a series of reactions designed to maintain homoestasis (Selye 1983). The model has undergone further refinement since it was originally proposed, but essentially describes three sequential stages (see Fig. 6.1). The initial response to the stressor is the alarm reaction and involves mobilization of the sympathetic nervous system and the release of hormones from the adrenal medulla in the fight and flight reaction. In this first phase, the adrenal cortex secretes increased amounts of glucocorticoids, including cortisol. This short-term response aims to help the individual cope with or adapt to the stressor and achieve homeostasis. If the threat continues then the person goes into the second stage of resistance or adaptation in which the adrenal cortex

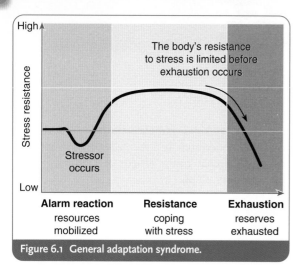

High

Stress resistance

The body's resistance to stress is limited before exhaustion occurs

Stressor occurs

Low

| **Alarm reaction** | **Resistance** | **Exhaustion** |
| resources mobilized | coping with stress | reserves exhausted |

Figure 6.1 General adaptation syndrome.

The three stages of the general adaptation syndrome occur sequentially and represent the body's response to stress which is mediated by changing levels of hormones, especially adrenaline and cortisol.

and medulla return to their usual rate of secreting hormones. These first two stages of the stress syndrome occur many times during our lives and we successfully adapt and cope. However, if there is continued exposure to the stressful situation then glucocorticoid secretion continues, but eventually decreases and there is a loss of resistance to stress. If this happens, the body is no longer able to cope and enters the final stage of exhaustion, ultimately leading to death (Selye 1983).

Physiology of stress response

The brain recognizes, evaluates and organizes the response to the stressor. The size and duration of the response is tailored to the particular characteristics of the stressor. Variations in responses result from individual differences in coping (Brunner 1997). In response to a stressor the brain influences the activity of all organs in the body via activation of the hypothalamic–pituitary–adrenal axis and the sympathetic–adreno-medullary system.

The hypothalamus is significant in the control of all aspects of the stress response. Corticotrophin-releasing hormone (CRH), produced in the hypothalamus, is instrumental in the activation of the stress response (O'Connor et al 2000). CRH is also secreted by neurons as a neurotransmitter. Such neurons from the hypothalamus project to areas in the brain stem that control the sympathetic nervous system and also to the locus coeruleus, another region in the brain stem (Lovallo 1997). Noradrenaline-secreting (noradrenergic) neurons arise in the locus coeruleus and project to the spinal cord, cerebellum, the hypothalamus and medulla oblongata. The CRH neurons and noradrenergic neurons in the brain form a positive feedback loop in the stress response system (O'Connor et al 2000).

The outcome of this reinforcing loop is that the hypothalamus activates mechanisms to prepare the body for flight or fight in the initial response to a stressful situation. Hypothalamic neurons project directly to autonomic regions in the spinal cord (DiMicco et al 2002). Sympathetic nerve impulses are transmitted from the spinal cord and lead to increases in heart rate, blood pressure and cardiac output, and also dilate large muscular arteries and the bronchioles. Sympathetic impulses also mobilize energy by provoking rises in blood glucose, glycerol and fatty acids (see Fig. 6.2). Adrenaline secretion from the adrenal medulla is stimulated by sympathetic impulses. Adrenaline enhances the magnitude of response and duration of effects of the sympathetic stimulation.

In addition to the metabolic and physiological changes just outlined, the secretion of adrenaline from the adrenal medulla and noradrenaline from sympathetic synapses enhances alertness and makes the individual more vigilant; both attributes are useful in dealing with a threat (Brunner 1997).

Hypothalamic CRH mediates the physiological responses to stress and is important in the activation of the sympathetic nervous system (Rothwell 1990) and the pituitary–adrenal axis. The secretion of nearly all hormones is altered during stress, but cortisol is especially important. In this acute stage of stress the hypothalamic–pituitary–adrenal axis (HPA axis) is activated (see Fig. 6.3). The stressor continues to stimulate the release of CRH from the hypothalamus, which in turn stimulates the secretion of adrenocorticotrophic hormone (ACTH) by the anterior pituitary gland. ACTH enters the general circulation and acts on the adrenal cortex to stimulate the release of glucocorticoids, mainly cortisol. Cortisol is carried in blood to many target tissues where it promotes increases in the levels of glucose, fatty acids and amino acids in the blood. ACTH is the most important trigger for the secretion of cortisol from the adrenal cortex, although other hormones, cytokines and autonomic nerve impulses may also control cortisol secretion (Tsigos & Chrousos 2002).

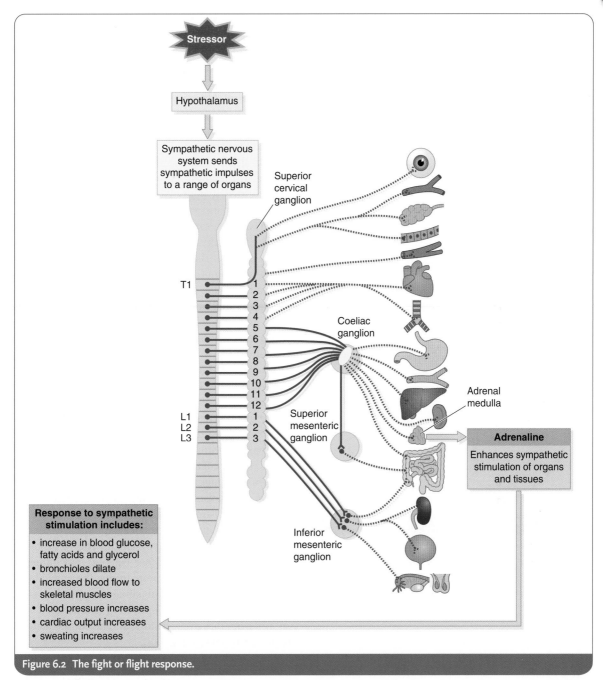

Figure 6.2 The fight or flight response.

During the alarm reaction stress activates the sympathetic nervous system which produces the fight or flight response enabling the individual to cope with an emergency. Sympathetic nerve impulses arriving at the adrenal medulla stimulate increased adrenaline secretion which enhances the sympathetic effects. (Adapted by kind permission from Waugh & Grant 2001.)

Once glucocorticoids are secreted via the HPA axis they feedback negatively on the hypothalamus to stop the release of CRH. This in turn leads to less ACTH and cortisol being secreted. The levels of cortisol and other glucocorticoids are usually kept within controlled boundaries (Miller and O'Callaghan 2002). In a non-stressed state, CRH is secreted in a series of short bursts, about three times an hour with increased secretion early in the

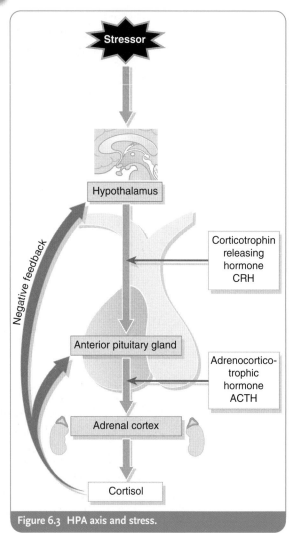

Figure 6.3 HPA axis and stress.

The brain perceives a stressful situation and sends messages to the hypothalamus. The HPA axis is activated, resulting in increased cortisol secretion from the adrenal cortex. Cortisol has a key role in mediating the stress response.

to endure a coexistence with pathogens (Selye 1983). Ultimately, via the negative feeback loops described, cortisol and the other glucocorticoids limit the duration of the stress response.

The body's adaptation to a stressor is mainly mediated by hormones. Many hormones such as cortisol, growth hormone and glucagon tend to raise blood glucose levels so that cells can produce enough energy to cope with the effects of the stressors. The secretion of antidiuretic hormone and aldosterone secretion are increased to raise the extracellular fluid volume to cope with potential haemorrhage caused by injury. An increase in metabolic rate is stimulated by increases in thyroid-stimulating hormone and thyroid hormones. Gonadotrophin secretion is inhibited to reduce fertility and increased growth hormone secretion also facilitates tissue growth and repair to cope with trauma. The renin–angiotensin system also plays a role in the stress response, renin secretion from the kidney and angiotensin-converting enzyme in the lungs produce angiotensin II, a powerful vasoconstrictor which increases blood pressure and heart rate (Black & Garbutt 2002).

The body's ability to adapt to stress or its 'adaptation energy' is finite. The stress response is designed to be limited such that the physiological responses mediated by the glucocorticoids are beneficial rather than harmful (Tsigos & Chrousos 2002). In the short term, the metabolic and immunosuppressive effects are homeostatic. However, if the stress response continues, exhaustion ensues, signalling that the body's homeostatic control mechanisms have failed. Prolonged stress leads to chronic problems, including tiredness, lack of energy, disturbed sleep, gastrointestinal symptoms, mental dysfunction and depression (von Onciul 1996). Exposure to stress during childhood (see Fig. 6.4) may influence brain development and programme the individual's responsiveness to stressful situations (Teicher et al 2003). Childhood social deprivation is associated with an 'unfavourable stress history' and health inequalities (Brunner 1997) (see Fig. 6.4).

morning. During stress, the secretion of CRH, ACTH and cortisol increases significantly (Tsigos & Chrousos 2002).

Glucocorticoids have many effects in addition to mobilizing energy, they control the whole body's response to stress and they suppress reproductive, growth and thyroid functions by inhibiting the anterior pituitary hormones, gonadotrophins, growth hormone and thyroid-stimulating hormone (Tsigos & Chrousos 2002). The glucocorticoids suppress immune responses, including inflammation, which enables the individual

Stress and disease

Chronic stress is thought to contribute to disease in a number of complex ways (Brunner 1997), since in prolonged stress levels of hormones are raised and homeostatic disturbances continue. Chronic psychosocial stress, such as bereavement, pressure at work and low socio-economic status, is a risk factor for chronic

Western societies and is characterized by the formation of plaques. Atherosclerosis is a generalized condition, affecting the large- and medium-sized arteries throughout the body. The process appears to begin as early as the teens, but since it progresses slowly, symptoms are rarely apparent until over 20 years later. The significance of atherosclerosis is that it impairs blood flow by narrowing or obstructing the lumen of the blood vessels. The plaques predispose to thrombus (clot) formation, which also obstructs the lumen (see Fig. 6.5). Clots that block small blood vessels supplying the heart cause heart attacks and those that block blood flow to the brain cause strokes. Thrombi can give rise to emboli (small fragments that break away from the clot), which can occlude the lumen of smaller 'downstream' vessels.

Inflammation plays a role in mediating the disease through all its stages (Libby et al 2002). The inner lining of the artery, called the endothelium, is crucial in maintaining the appropriate muscle tone of the vessel; this is achieved by chemicals produced in the endothelium. These chemicals stop clots forming and prevent platelets adhering to the vessel lining (de Belder 1993).

There are many events that contribute to the atherosclerotic process. One of the key changes that occurs in the formation of atherosclerotic lesions is the binding of white blood cells to the endothelium and their infiltration into the intima of the arterial wall. The binding of white blood cells is due to the appearance of specific adhesion molecules that bind certain types of white blood cells, specifically monocytes, macrophages and lymphocytes (Libby et al 2002). The adhesion molecules only appear following endothelial damage and this may be due to elevated levels of cholesterol and triglycerides in the blood, high blood pressure and tobacco smoke (de Belder 1993). Following their infiltration into the intima, the white blood cells contribute to the inflammatory response. The macrophages scavenge and ingest lipid and develop

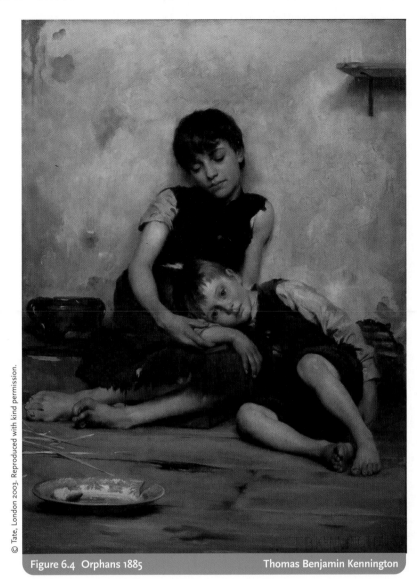

Figure 6.4 Orphans 1885   Thomas Benjamin Kennington

illness (Pickering 2001). In particular, chronic stress is implicated in the aetiology and pathogenesis of cardiovascular diseases, including atherosclerosis (Black & Garbutt 2002). Stress is also associated with the onset or exacerbation of symptoms in many chronic disorders of the gastrointestinal tract, including inflammatory bowel disease and peptic ulcer disease (Mayer 2000). Psychosocial stress also contributes to morbidity among individuals with asthma and may also be a risk factor in the pathogenesis of the disease (Wright et al 1998).

Stress and cardiovascular disease

Stress plays a major role in the development of atherosclerosis. Atherosclerosis is a common disease in

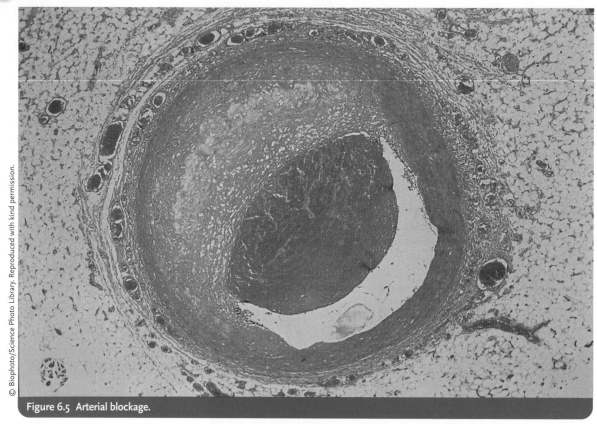

Figure 6.5 Arterial blockage.

Light micrograph of a section through a human coronary artery showing the almost total obstruction of the lumen by the development of a haemorrhage (bright red) into an atheromatous plaque.

into foam cells (Libby et al 2002). Platelets also become activated by the endothelial damage and adhere to the site of inflammation. The cells that have infiltrated the intima accumulate and divide and fat builds up within them; fibrous tissue also forms within the intima (Black & Garbutt 2002). The plaques formed typically consist of a core of lipid (mainly cholesterol) covered by a fibrous cap (smooth muscle and connective tissue).

All these changes lead to the thickening of the artery wall and a diminution in the size of the lumen. As the plaque grows, it may give rise to symptoms of reduced blood flow, such as angina or claudication (pain in the legs on walking). If the lesion is disrupted, a fissure can occur in the plaque, which promotes the formation of a thrombus. Over time these thrombi can accumulate within the atherosclerotic lesion and can completely occlude the vessel (de Belder 1993).

It appears that the process of atherosclerosis is an exaggerated and prolonged inflammatory reaction. Risk factors such as high blood pressure and free radicals from smoking make the endothelium more prone to damage and fat cells produce inflammatory chemicals. The inflamed endothelium attracts macrophages and lymphocytes; once these cells have stuck and squeezed through the endothelial cells they release inflammatory chemicals that attack muscle cells. Inflammatory signals then cause both the macrophages and muscle cells to engulf cholesterol. Plaques that are more inflamed are likely to form clots that lead to heart attacks and strokes (Phillips 2003). Appreciating that inflammation is central to the process of atherosclerosis explains why infections may increase the risk of cardiovascular disease (Phillips 2003). Microorganisms such as herpes viruses and *Chlamydia pneumoniae* may stimulate the release of inflammatory chemicals that may irritate the endothelium and provoke atherosclerosis (Libby 2002).

The suggestion is that recurrent stress can initiate and promote atherosclerosis. Stress promotes endothelial damage, the appearance of adhesion molecules and the activation of macrophages and foam cell formation. The mediators of the stress response, including corticosteroids, initiate atherosclerosis and lead to its progression. Stress leads to changes in the lipid profile of blood consistent with atherosclerosis. Lipids are transported in plasma by lipoproteins. LDL (low density lipoprotein) is the main carrier of cholesterol, and high concentrations in the plasma increase the risk of atherosclerosis, whereas high density lipoprotein (HDL) is protective (Libby 2002). LDL passes through the endothelium and becomes oxidized once trapped in the artery wall. Modified LDL participates in the formation of foam cells and therefore plaque formation. Stress contributes to the oxidation of lipids and to the inflammatory response, leading to atherosclerosis (Black & Garbutt 2002).

In contrast, the beneficial effects of moderate amounts of alcohol on reducing the risk of coronary heart disease probably relates in part to its effects on blood lipid transport and a reduction in the deposition of cholesterol in the walls of blood vessels (Klatsky 2003). Aspirin, a non-steroidal anti-inflammatory drug, is also protective against ischaemic heart disease. This is considered to be due to aspirin's ability to reduce clotting factors and vasoconstriction rather than due to its anti-inflammatory effects (Pacini 1997, Libby 2002).

Stress and the immune system

The links between stress, the immune system and an individual's health are widely accepted. Psychological stress associated with stressful life events is linked to increased susceptibility to illness, including infections (Stone et al 1992, Yang & Glaser 2002). It is also hypothesized that psychological stress predisposes individuals to allergies and cancers by suppressing immune function (Tomatis 2001).

Psychoneuroimmunology is the field of study that provides a framework for examining the interrelationships between the nervous, endocrine and immune systems and an exploration of the clinical and therapeutic implications (Yang & Glaser 2002). The mind–body links are emphasized in psychoneuroimmunology, making it particularly relevant to healthcare (Schrader 1996). Psychoneuroimmunology reinforces both the holistic nature of health and the holistic approach to care.

If there is a connection between emotions, thoughts, experiences and attitudes and an individual's immune response, then the links need to be identified. The mind–body interrelationship relies on the bi-directional flow of hormones, neurotransmitters and cytokines (see Fig. 6.6) (Blalock 1984, Haddad et al 2002). Autonomic nerve fibres connect to lymphoid organs including the

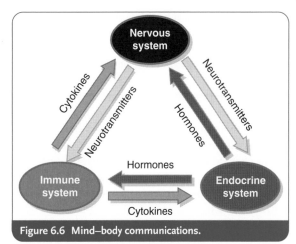

Figure 6.6 Mind–body communications.

Communication between the three systems is possible because of the overlapping roles of hormones, neurotransmitters and cytokines and the existence of receptors in each system capable of responding to these signals.

thymus and spleen, and cells of the immune system such as lymphocytes have receptors for neurotransmitters and hormones. This illustrates that the nervous and endocrine systems are capable of modulating the immune system (Felten 1991, Schorr & Arnason 1999, Yang & Glaser 2002). Immune cells in turn can be stimulated to secrete cytokines that trigger the hypothalamus to produce CRH and the activation of the HPA axis (Haddad et al 2002). The interrelationships between neurological, endocrine and immunological cells are possible because they possess receptors enabling them to respond to each other's chemical signals.

The alteration of immune function by stressors is thought to be mediated by the sympathetic adreno-medullary system in acute stress and by the HPA axis in more long-term stress (O'Leary et al 1996). Prolonged activity of the HPA axis in stress is associated with immunosuppression and negative influences on health (O'Leary 1990). For example, examination stress suppresses and enhances various aspects of immune function (Maes et al 1997) and psychological stress is considered to delay wound healing because it disturbs immune aspects of the healing process (Kiecolt-Glaser et al 1995). Dysregulation of the immune system by psychological stress can make individuals more susceptible to infections (Stone et al 1992, Yang & Glaser 2002).

Corticosteroids are considered to be the principal mediators in the immunosuppressive effect of stress (Buckingham 1998). Immunosuppression is thought to be due to apoptosis (programmed cell death) in lymphocytes and the repression of genes necessary for producing an effective immune response (Auphan et al 1996). Inhibition of cytokine production by immune cells also contributes to immunosuppression (O'Connor et al 2000).

Whilst immune function is modulated by the nervous and endocrine systems, challenges to the immune system can in turn influence the nervous and endocrine systems (Anisman et al 1996). Chronic fatigue syndrome has a complex and multifactorial aetiology and viral illnesses may be one of many risk factors in this heterogeneous condition (Jackson 2002, Afari & Buchwald 2003).

In summary, psychological stressors can lead to changes in immune function and are associated with detrimental effects on health. These effects are mediated by chemical signals and receptors linking the nervous, endocrine and immune systems.

Stress and cancer

There is a great deal of controversy over whether there is a positive association between stressful life events and cancer. Adding to this controversy is the suggestion that there is a preoccupation with demonstrating that stressful life events are linked to cancer (McGee 1999). This could be linked to the notion that 'Theories that diseases are caused by mental states and can be cured by will power are always an index of how much is not understood about the physical terrain of a disease' (Sontag 1991). In the 1970s, when this was first written, Sontag suggested that the mythology of cancer incorporated the view that repression of feelings was the cause of cancer. Sontag suggests that the metaphors of cancer including 'killer disease' and 'cancer victims' and the psychological theories make the cancer patient responsible for both 'falling ill and getting well'. Views of cancer have changed in the last 30 years (Tomatis 2001), but there is still a stigma associated with the diagnosis of cancer. More recently, in a collection of e-mails published after her death from breast cancer, Ruth Picardie wrote 'Cancer is all about fear, secrecy and euphemism- palliative care, advanced disease – all are euphemisms for dying. Oncology is the biggest euphemism in the world' (Picardie 1998).

The role of stressful events and breast cancer has been widely studied (Tomatis 2001), although there is no consensus yet over the possible correlation between psychological stress and breast cancer. A report of a study examining the relationship between adverse life events and breast cancer suggests that women with breast cancer experience more severe life events in the five years preceding diagnosis (Chen et al 1995). The biological mechanism that could explain this suggested association has yet to be elucidated, but may result from stress-induced changes in immune surveillance enabling undetected cancer cells to multiply. The authors of this study do acknowledge that other mechanisms may account for their findings and suggest that longer prospective studies are needed (Chen et al 1995). In a study that set out to replicate the findings of Chen et al (1995), no support for the theory that severe life events may be implicated in the cause of breast cancer was found (Protheroe et al 1999). The disparity in findings amongst such studies is possibly partly due to methodological problems and the lack of clearly articulated hypotheses being tested (McGee 1999).

Stress and mental illness

Psychological stress is implicated in both the onset and development of mental illness, including schizophrenia, anxiety disorders and depression (Herbert 1997). The evidence that links life events to depression is most compelling. Possible mechanisms for stress-induced mental illness remain to be elucidated, although stress hormones such as CRH and cortisol are known to exert effects on neuronal function in the brain (O'Connor et al 2000). Changes in hormones resulting from stress may also regulate monoamines (Herbert 1997). Monoamines such as dopamine, noradrenaline and serotonin are implicated in the development and course of depression (Nemeroff 1998). Prolonged activity in the HPA axis, especially the increased secretion of CRH, is considered significant in depression (Nemeroff 1998, Dinan 2001). The dysfunction of the CRH-secreting neurons in the hypothalamus is thought to be key to the chronic hyperactivity that develops in the HPA axis, and to the onset of depression.

In a model that attempts to link childhood stress to depression in later life, abuse or neglect in childhood activates the stress response and triggers sustained activity in the CRH-secreting neurons in the brain. These neurons may become sensitized if the stress and therefore hyperactivity persist. Permanent changes occur in the developing brain due to this increased CRH activity that make an individual more susceptible to depression in adulthood (Nemeroff 1998).

To summarize, the response to stress involves a coordinated array of biochemical signals including hormones, neurotransmitters and cytokines that strive to promote homeostasis. There are two main limbs to the neuroendocrine response to stressors. The fight or flight response involves the sympathetic and adrenomedullary systems, which prime the body for action. The slower and more prolonged response to stress involves the HPA axis and results in the secretion of glucocorticoids, such as cortisol, from the adrenal cortex. Cortisol elicits a variety of effects that enable the individual to withstand prolonged exposure to stressors. Chronic stress is implicated in the aetiology and pathogenesis of many diseases, some of which have been highlighted.

Introducing the autonomic nervous system

The autonomic nervous system (ANS) is part of the peripheral nervous system (PNS) and is traditionally described as the motor division that controls visceral (internal) organs. However, the ANS does have sensory receptors and sensory neurons; sensory input to the ANS comes via the visceral afferent system and the somatic afferent system (Pacini 1999). The major role of the autonomic system is to control internal functions that are not usually under conscious control, in order to maintain a relatively stable internal environment. The ANS sends motor neurons to muscles in the heart, smooth muscle in internal organs such as the intestine, bladder and uterus, and to secretory glands.

Sympathetic and parasympathetic divisions

The ANS is split into two subdivisions. The sympathetic nervous system is involved in the fight or flight response helping the body to cope with stressful situations. The parasympathetic nervous system is active when the body is operating under ambient conditions; it is involved in relaxation. Both systems innervate the same organs and usually act in opposition to maintain homeostasis. Although the description as 'autonomic' suggests that this division is 'self-governing' the ANS is actually regulated by parts of the brain, including the hypothalamus and medulla oblongata (Pacini 1999).

The arrangement of the neurons in the sympathetic nervous system (SNS) and parasympathetic nervous system (PSNS) is different in a number of respects. The neurons of the SNS arise from the neck, thorax and abdominal regions of the spinal cord; the cervical, thoracic and lumbar outflows. The neurons of the PSNS arise from the brain and form some of the cranial nerves including the vagus nerve (cranial nerve X); in addition there is an outflow from the sacral region of the spinal cord (see Fig. 6.7).

Structure of pathways

Motor neurons in the autonomic nervous system do not reach their effectors or targets directly, as those motor neurons in the somatic division do, but rather connect to a secondary motor neuron that in turn innervates the target organ. The two neurons in the pathway to the effector form a synapse in one of the ganglia outside the central nervous system. These autonomic ganglia contain collections of cell bodies and dendrites. The first neuron in the pathway to the effector organ is called the preganglionic neuron. The cell body of this neuron is located in either the brain stem or spinal cord. In the ganglion the axon terminal of the preganglionic fibre forms a synapse with the dendrites of the second neuron in the pathway, the postganglionic neuron. Nerve impulses are transmitted from the preganglionic neuron to the postganglionic neuron via chemical neurotransmitters in the process of synaptic transmission (see Ch. 5). The postganglionic neuron begins in a ganglion and its axon connects to either cardiac muscle, smooth muscle or a secretory gland (see Fig. 6.7). These neurons connect to muscle cells via neuromuscular junctions (see Ch. 5). The preganglionic fibre is myelinated just like somatic motor neurons are, whilst the postganglionic fibres are unmyelinated.

In addition to the distinguishing features noted, there are a number of other differences in the arrangement of neurons and chemical transmitter substances in the two divisions of the ANS. The ganglia of the SNS lie close to the CNS whilst the ganglia of the PSNS are distributed in the tissues of the effector organ. This means that in the SNS the preganglionic fibre is short and the postganglionic fibre long, whilst in the PSNS the opposite situation exists.

Autonomic neurotransmitters and receptors

The chemical transmitter substance secreted by the preganglionic fibres in both divisions is acetylcholine (Ach). Postganglionic fibres of the SNS secrete noradrenaline and are called adrenergic neurons, and in the PSNS the postganglionic fibres secrete Ach and are called cholinergic neurons (see Fig. 6.7) (Pacini 1999).

The difference in effects of parasympathetic and sympathetic impulses on target organs is due to the

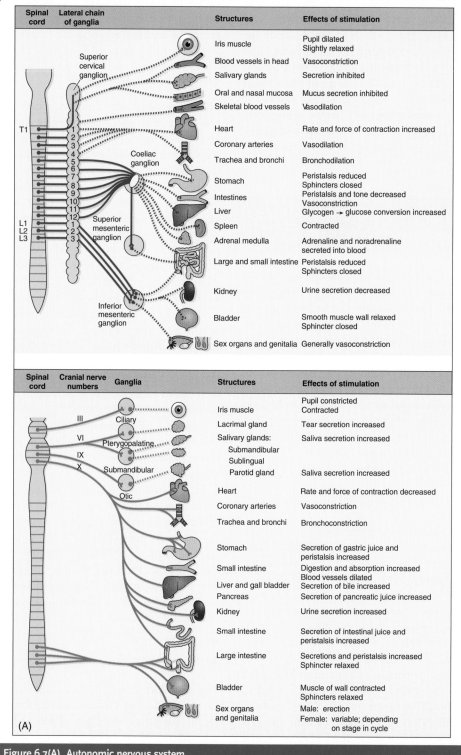

Figure 6.7(A) Autonomic nervous system.

(A) The major autonomic pathways are shown, illustrating that the sympathetic fibres arise in the thoracic and lumbar regions of the spinal cord whilst the parasympathetic pathways begin in the brain or sacral region of the spinal cord. Each pathway consists of a pre- and a postganglionic fibre. (Reproduced with kind permission from Waugh & Grant 2001.)

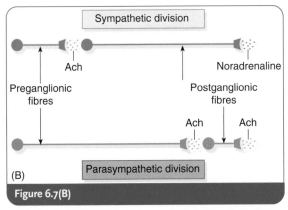

Figure 6.7(B)

(B) Both sympathetic and parasympathetic preganglionic fibres secrete acetylcholine (Ach). Sympathetic postganglionic fibres secrete noradrenaline whilst parasympathetic postganglionic fibres secrete Ach.

different chemicals, acetylcholine and noradrenaline, and their receptors. For example, noradrenaline secreted by the arrival of sympathetic impulses at the sinoatrial node causes the heart to beat faster, whilst acetylcholine secretion resulting from parasympathetic impulses causes the heart rate to slow.

Each neurotransmitter has a number of specialized receptor sub-types; noradrenaline has four types of receptor with slightly different shapes; alpha receptors (α_1 and α_2) and beta receptors (β_1 and β_2). Two main classes of acetylcholine receptors are identified on the basis of their responsiveness to nicotine or the toadstool alkaloid, muscarine.

Both noradrenaline and adrenaline (the hormone from the adrenal medulla) can stimulate adrenergic receptors on effector cells. Noradrenaline mainly combines with alpha receptors whereas adrenaline can combine with either type of receptor. The effect of these adrenergic substances on effectors depends on the relative proportions of alpha and beta receptors. The responses of adrenergic receptors can be excitatory or inhibitory. There are a number of adrenergic receptor types found in different target organs. Alpha 1 receptors are found in the smooth muscle of most arterioles and in sphincter muscles of the gastrointestinal tract and bladder, whilst alpha 2 receptors are found in parts of the GI tract. The dominant type of receptors in the heart are beta 1 receptors. Beta 2 receptors are found in the bronchioles of the lung, the wall muscles of the bladder, arterioles of skeletal muscles, brain and lung, and some parts of the gastrointestinal tract (Rang et al 1999).

Because of the difference in neurotransmitters and their receptor sub-types many different drugs have been developed that act selectively to stimulate or inhibit autonomic transmission. Drugs that stimulate receptors are called agonists and those that inhibit receptors are called antagonists, or blockers. Drugs called beta blockers were originally developed for the treatment of high blood pressure. Because they literally 'block' the beta receptors, noradrenaline cannot interact with beta receptors in the heart, so the heart beats more slowly and, because the heart pumps less blood, the blood pressure will fall. Unfortunately, because there are beta receptors in other target organs, including bronchioles, beta blockers have unwanted side effects such as narrowing the air passages (bronchoconstriction) making it more difficult to breathe.

As drugs have become more sophisticated they are more selective, so modern beta blockers such as atenolol will only block the beta 1 receptors in the heart and not beta 2 receptors in the bronchioles as earlier beta blockers did (Pacini 1999). Not only are beta blockers effective in reducing morbidity and mortality in individuals with hypertension (Philipp et al 1997), but they are also used in the management of heart failure. The use of beta blockers has been shown in several controlled trials to improve the prognosis and to reduce hospital admissions in individuals with symptomatic congestive heart failure (Gibbs et al 2000, Packer et al 2001).

Drugs that selectively bind to beta 2 receptors in bronchioles relax the smooth muscle and dilate the bronchioles. Inhaled beta 2 agonist bronchodilators, such as salbutamol, are integral components of effective asthma treatment since the bronchodilation makes breathing easier (Busse 1996).

There are two main types of postsynaptic receptor that bind acetylcholine. Acetylcholine receptors stimulated by nicotine (the chemical found in tobacco smoke, which is addictive) are called nicotinic receptors and are found in the autonomic ganglia. When stimulated, these receptors produce rapid excitatory responses. The acetylcholine receptors stimulated by muscarine are called muscarinic receptors and are found in effector organs (Pacini 1999). Responses from these receptors are also excitatory, but occur relatively slowly. Muscarine is a toxin found in a number of mushrooms, although it was discovered in *Amanita muscari,* hence its name. Muscarine causes symptoms that mimic parasympathetic stimulation and include excessive salivation, sweating, tears, abdominal cramps and visual disturbances (Pacini 1999). Atropine is an anticholinergic drug that blocks muscarinic receptors in effector organs. It has various effects on different target organs, including relaxation of the gut wall and dilatation of pupils. Atropine is also used as a premedication prior to anaesthesia because it decreases bronchial and salivary secretions.

Having emphasized the crucial role that noradrenaline and acetylcholine play in the effects of sympathetic and parasympathetic postganglionic impulses on their effector organ, it is recognized that other neurotransmitters may also be involved. Both sympathetic and parasympathetic postganglionic neurons are also able to secrete additional transmitter substances in a process called cotransmission. A combination of neurotransmitters being released from a single neuron has the ability to produce a variety of responses in the effector tissue (Lundberg 1996, Pacini 1999).

Summary

The autonomic nervous system has an enormous role to play in maintaining the body's internal environment within tolerable limits. The two divisions of the autonomic nervous system have different effects on their target organs, but both contribute to homeostasis. The sympathetic nervous system is an important mediator of the 'fight or flight' response in stressful situations, whilst the parasympathetic nervous system is active during relaxation, helping to conserve energy. Noradrenaline and acetylcholine are the neurotransmitters secreted from the sympathetic and parasympathetic postganglionic motor neurons and they account for the different effects on target organs. Each of these neurotransmitters interacts with a number of specialized receptor sub-types. Noradrenaline combines with beta and alpha adrenergic receptors, whilst acetylcholine combines with muscarinic receptors in target organs. Many drugs have been developed that can either stimulate or block these receptors and they play a crucial role in the treatment of a variety of conditions.

References

Afari N, Buchwald D 2003 Chronic fatigue syndrome: a review. American Journal of Psychiatry 160(2):221–236

Anisman H, Baines M G, Berczi I et al 1996 Neuroimmune mechanisms in health and disease: 2. Disease. Canadian Medical Association Journal 155(8):1075–1082

Auphan N, Didonato J A, Helmberg A et al 1996 Immunoregulatory genes and immunosuppression by glucocorticoids. Toxicology Letters 88:3

Black P H, Garbutt L D 2002 Stress, inflammation and cardiovascular disease. Journal of Psychosomatic Research 52(1):1–23

Blalock J E 1984 The immune system as a sensory organ. Journal of Immunology 133:1067–1070

Brunner E 1997 Socioeconomic determinants of health: stress and the biology of inequality. British Medical Journal 314(7092):1472–1476

Buckingham J C 1998 Stress and the neuroendocrine-immune axis. Pathophysiology 5(Supplement 1):144

Busse W W 1996 Long- and short-acting beta2-adrenergic agonists. Effects on airway function in patients with asthma. Archives of Internal Medicine 156(14):1514–1520

Chen C C, David A S, Nunnerley H et al 1995 Adverse life events and breast cancer: case-control study. British Medical Journal 311:1527–1530

Cooper C L 1992 Stress management. Biological Sciences Review 5(2):27–29

de Belder A 1993 Understanding atherosclerosis. Nursing Standard 7(30):48–49

DiMicco J A, Samuels B C, Zaretskaia M V et al 2002 The dorsomedial hypothalamus and the response to stress. Pharmacology and Behaviour 71(3):469–480

Dinan T G 2001 Psychoneuroendocrinology of mood disorders. Current Opinion in Psychiatry 14(1):51–55

Felten D L 1991 Neurotransmitter signalling of cells of the immune system: important progress, major gaps. Brain, Behaviour and Immunity 5:2–8

Gibbs C R, Davies M K, Lip G Y H 2000 Management: digoxin and other inotropes, β blockers, and antiarrhythmic and antithrombotic treatment. British Medical Journal 320:495–498

Haddad J J, Saadé N E, Safieh-Garabedian B 2002 Cytokines and neuro-immune-endocrine interactions: a role for the hypothalamic-pituitary-adrenal revolving axis. Journal of Neuroimmunology 133(1–2):1–19

Herbert J 1997 Stress, the brain and mental illness. British Medical Journal 315:530–535

Jackson E 2002 An overview of chronic fatigue syndrome. Nursing Standard 17(13):45–53

Kiecolt-Glaser J K, Marucha P T, Malarkey W B et al 1995 Slowing of wound healing by psychological stress. Lancet 346:1194–1196

Klatsky A L 2003 Drink to your health? Scientific American 288(3):62–69

Lazarus R S, Folkman S 1984 Stress, appraisal, and coping. Springer, New York

Libby P 2002 Atherosclerosis: the new view. Scientific American 286(5):30–37

Libby P, Ridker P M, Maseri A 2002 Inflammation and atherosclerosis. Circulation 105(9):1135–1143

Lovallo W R 1997 Stress & health biological and psychological interactions. Sage Publications, London

Lundberg J M 1996 Pharmacology of cotransmission in the autonomic nervous system: integrative aspects on amines, neuropeptides, adenosine triphopshate, amino acids and nitric oxide. Pharmacology Review 48(1):113–178

Maes M, Song C, Lin A et al 1997 The effects of psychological stress on the immune system in humans. Biological Psychiatry 42(1) Supplement 1:5S

Mayer E A 2000 The neurobiology of stress and gastrointestinal disease. Gut 47(6):861–869

McGee R 1999 Does stress cause cancer? British Medical Journal 319:1015–1016

Miller D B, O'Callaghan J P 2002 Neuroendocrine aspects to stress. Metabolism 51(6 Part 2):5–10

Nemeroff C B 1998 The neurobiology of depression. Scientific American 278(6):28–35

O'Connor T M, O'Halloran D J, Shanahan F 2000 The stress response and the hypothalamic-pituitary-adrenal axis: from molecule to melancholia. Quarterly Journal of Medicine 93(6):323–333

O'Leary A 1990 Stress, emotion and human immune function. Psychology Bulletin 108:363–382

O'Leary A, Savard J, Miller S M 1996 Psychoneuroimmunology: elucidating the process. Current Opinion in Psychiatry 9(6): 427–432

Pacini D J 1997 An aspirin a day. Biological Sciences Review 10(1):25–29

Pacini D J 1999 The autonomic nervous system. Biological Sciences Review 11(4):30–34

Packer M, Coats A, Fowler M B et al 2001 Effect of carvedilol on survival in severe chronic heart failure. New England Journal of Medicine 344(22):1651–1658

Philipp T, Anlauf M, Distler A et al 1997 Randomised, double blind, multicentre comparison of hydrochloride, atenolol, nitrendipine, and enalapril in antihypertensive treatment: results of the HANE study. British Medical Journal 315:154–159

Phillips H 2003 Heart-stopping. New Scientist 177(2377):36–39

Picardie R 1998 Before I say goodbye. Penguin, Harmondsworth, p 13

Pickering T 2001 Job stress, control, and chronic disease: moving to the next level of evidence. Psychosomatic Medicine 63(5): 734–736

Protheroe D, Turvey K, Horgan K et al 1999 Stressful life events and difficulties and onset of breast cancer: case control study. British Medical Journal 319:1027–1030

Rang H P, Dale M M, Ritter J M 1999 Pharmacology, 4th edn. Churchill Livingstone, Edinburgh

Rice P L 1992 Stress & health, 2nd edn. Brookes/Cole, California

Rothwell N J 1990 Central effects of CRF on metabolism and energy balance. Neuroscience and Biobehavioral Reviews 14(3):263–271

Schorr E, Arnason B 1999 Interactions between the sympathetic nervous system and the immune system. Brain, Behaviour and Immunity 13:271–278

Schrader K A 1996 Stress and immunity after traumatic injury: the mind–body link. AACN Clinical Issue 7(3):351–358

Selye H 1983 The stress concept: past, present and future. In: Cooper C L (ed) Stress research issues for the eighties. John Wiley, Chichester, p 1–20

Sontag S 1991 Illness as metaphor and AIDS and its metaphors. Penguin, Harmondsworth, p 56

Stone A A, Bovbjerg D H, Neale J M et al 1992 Development of common cold symptoms following experimental rhinovirus infection is related to prior stressful life events. Behavioral Medicine 18:115–120

Teicher M H, Andersen S L, Polcari A et al 2003 The neurobiological consequences of early stress and childhood maltreatment. Neuroscience and Biobehavioral Reviews 27:33–44

Tomatis L 2001 Between the body and the mind the involvement of psychosocial factors in the development of multifactorial diseases. European Journal of Cancer 37(8):148–152

Tsigos C, Chrousos G P 2002 Hypothalamic-pituitary-adrenal axis, neuroendocrine factors and stress. Journal of Psychosomatic Research 53(4):865–871

von Onciul J 1996 ABC of work related disorder: stress at work. British Medical Journal 313(7059):745–748

Waugh A, Grant A 2001 Ross and Wilson: Anatomy and physiology in health and illness. Churchill Livingstone, Edinburgh

Wright R, Rodriguez M, Cohen S 1998 Review of psychosocial stress and asthma: an integrated biopsychosocial approach. Thorax 53(12):1066–1074

Yang E V, Glaser R 2002 Stress induced immunomodulation and implications for health. International Immunopharmacology 2(2–3):315–324

7

SLEEP

❝ But it was not the Lilac Fairy's intention to keep only Aurora safe, swaddled in dreamless sleep. She swept her wand over the heads of the courtiers and ladies-in-waiting, the princes and the guests, the King and Queen. And one by one they fell asleep where they stood or sat or sprawled or knelt, sinking into sleep like the leaves settling to the ground from an autumn tree. ❞

('The Sleeping Beauty', McCaughrean 1994)

Although sleep occupies a considerable portion of our lives no one really knows exactly why we need sleep. Sleep is a mysterious phenomenon that attracts inquiry from a diverse range of perspectives. Sleep is associated with rest and recuperation (Rodéhn Fox 1999) and anyone deprived of sleep for long periods becomes disturbed and unwell. Reflecting on the importance of sleep in our own lives overwhelmingly confirms that sleep is important for health, necessary for mental and physical wellbeing. Lack of sleep leaves us feeling tired and miserable, less able to concentrate or function properly. Sleep contributes to homeostasis, in the sense that without regular amounts of sleep, a sense of wellbeing is not achieved; any deficits in sleep also stimulate the body to obtain more sleep (Moorcroft 1993).

Although sleep research is now a burgeoning area of research, it is only in the last 50–70 years that much has been learned about sleep (Martensen 1995). Until the 1950s, sleep researchers thought that brain wave patterns were consistently slow during sleep. Rapid eye movement sleep (REM) was discovered in 1953 by Aserinsky and Kleitman and thought to be associated with dreaming. This led to a great interest in studying sleep, dreaming and sleep disorders in sleep laboratories and an increased understanding of the stages of sleep, together with the roles of the nervous and endocrine systems in sleep (Moorcroft 1993, Martensen 1995).

Sleep can be described in a number of ways, such as a temporary loss of consciousness, a state of unresponsiveness and inertia (Oswald 1966). Another explanation is that sleep is a regularly recurring suspension of consciousness that is reversible and more or less spontaneous. Sleep is characterized by a typical posture of closed eyes and reduced awareness of stimuli (see Fig. 7.1) (Donovan 1988). The recurrent pattern of sleeping and waking is the most obvious biological rhythm with a 24-hour cycle; these cycles are called circadian rhythms.

Keeping time: the rhythm of life

Rhythms are a feature of all organisms including humans; certain substances, processes and activities change in a rhythmic way. These rhythms and cycles are kept to time by biological timing systems that include 'stopwatches', 'clocks' and 'calendars' (Minors 1997, Young 2000, Wright 2002).

The biological timing system

Biological timepieces keep track of different intervals of time and with different degrees of precision, some are clusters of nerve cells in the brain and others are molecules (Wright 2002). The way in which the brain is able to measure time is still under speculation. It may be that our memories of events that filled a period of time help us to keep track of days, weeks, months and years. The brain seems to be able to measure the passage of seconds and minutes accurately, suggesting that there is a single internal reference clock (McCrone 1997).

The brain relies on split-second timing when coordinating muscle movements and the basal ganglia, which play a key role in controlling movement (see p. 66), are also thought to be involved in timing intervals of seconds to hours. The interval timer is thought to act like a stopwatch, but with a more complicated mechanism.

There are three components in this timepiece. The first is a group of neurons in the striatum located within the basal ganglia, called spiny neurons, which receive inputs from two sources that together start the stopwatch. The first part of the start signal comes from the substantia nigra, a group of neurons in the midbrain. Neurons from this area form synapses with the spiny neurons in the striatum; they secrete a burst of dopamine that signals the spiny neurons to start timing the pattern of impulses they are receiving from a group of cortical cells. These cortical cells are the third component in the

Figure 7.1 The Moon and Sleep 1894   Simeon Solomon

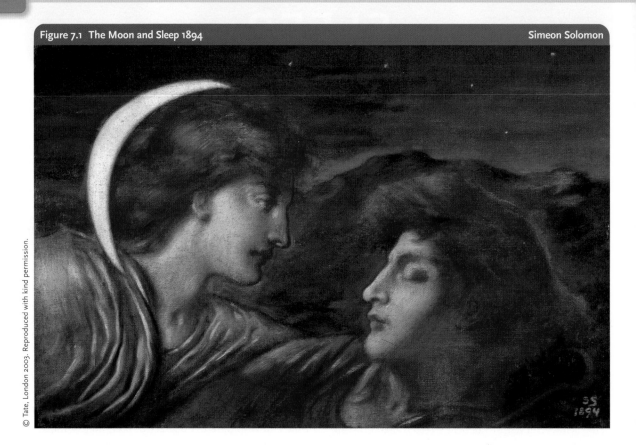

timepiece and they provide the second part of the start signal. When their attention is caught, they fire impulses in synchrony and the resulting spike acts like the pressing of a 'start button'. As they resume their usual pattern of firing, the cortical nerve impulses are monitored by the spiny neurons and once the familiar time intervals have elapsed, the stop switch is pressed and messages are sent via the thalamus to the cerebral cortex, where memories and decisions are made (Wright 2002).

The suggested time-keeping role of the dopamine-producing nerve cells of the substantia nigra is corroborated by findings that suggest that individuals with Parkinson's disease, whose neurons secrete less dopamine in the striatum, have problems measuring short intervals of time (McCrone 1997, Wright 2002). This interval timer is not particularly accurate, so for precision timing we rely on a circadian clock. This clock guides us to sleep at night and be awake during daylight as well as controlling many other core rhythms.

Experiments performed in which subjects had no access to light and dark cues resulted in the individuals adopting only a slightly longer cycle of about 25 hours. The fact that humans seem to keep good time suggests

that other cues, social factors and zeitgebers (German for 'time giver') are important in their sleep–wake cycle (Donovan 1988). The observation that individuals deprived of usual light and darkness cycles continue to display circadian rhythms also suggests that there is an endogenous mechanism that generates the 24-hour rhythm (Dijk 1996). In humans the 'biological clock' that dictates the day–night cycle of activity, the circadian rhythm, is located in the suprachiasmatic nuclei (SCN) in the hypothalamus (see Fig. 7.2) (Young 2000).

Since circadian patterns continue irrespective of daylight, light is not necessary to establish circadian rhythms (Wright 2002). However, light is important for time-keeping since it synchronizes the rhythmic activity of the SCN and entrains the circadian clock to the daylight and night-time cycles (Wright 2002).

Experiments with fruit flies in the 1960s and 1970s revealed the presence of 'clock' genes that have a sense of time (Weiner 1999). Clock genes within the SCN are switched on and off by the proteins they code for in a feedback loop with a 24-hour rhythm. These 'clock gene' rhythms are intrinsic and self-perpetuating without any light, dark or other exogenous cues. Light helps to

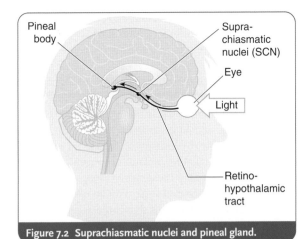

Figure 7.2 Suprachiasmatic nuclei and pineal gland.

The SCN receives impulses from the retina about the brightness and duration of light. This information is passed to the pineal gland where melatonin secretion is suppressed by light.

synchronize the rhythms of activity of clock genes to match the prevailing environmental pattern. Clock genes produce proteins that in turn control further genetic pathways influencing physiological activity and homeostasis (Young 2000). Intriguingly, clock genes are found widely dispersed in the body, suggesting that other organs and tissues also display circadian rhythmicity (Wright 2002).

Circadian rhythms

There are many examples of circadian rhythms, including body temperature, which oscillates around a set point, the secretion of certain hormones, urine output and cardiovascular functions (Clancy & McVicar 1994a, Wright 2002). In addition, certain pathophysiological events relate to the circadian phase: asthma attacks are more common around 04.00, cerebrovascular accidents frequently occur around 08.00 and pain may be at its worst around 21.00 (Young 2000). Many cardiac disorders, including chest pain and heart attacks, occur more frequently at two times of the day: around midnight and in the early morning 06.30–08.30 (Thompson 1992).

Many physiological rhythms influence or are influenced by sleep (Moorcroft 1993). Circadian rhythms are important for health (Clancy & McVicar 1994a), any desynchronization, such as night work or hospitalization, may have an adverse effect on mental and physical wellbeing (Clancy & McVicar 1994b, Baxendale

et al 1997). Some of the negative effects can be reversed by having short periods of sleep during a night shift, since this helps to stabilize circadian rhythms (Waterhouse & Minors 1993). Flying across time zones also causes desynchronization of circadian rhythms and a range of symptoms commonly known as 'jet lag'. The severity of the symptoms is directly related to the number of time zones which are crossed. These problems arise due to the mismatch between the body clock and exogenous cues (Waterhouse & Minors 1993). Jet lag may also be attributed to the 'lagging behind' of circadian rhythmicity in other organs and tissues, and whilst the SCN will be reset by the new light–dark cycle, it may take longer for all the organs to resynchronize (Wright 2002).

Sleep–wake cycle and sleep cycles

Sleep could be described as the physically inactive part of the circadian sleep–wake activity cycle. However, much brain activity occurs during sleep and this can be measured by the electroencephalogram (EEG). Electrodes attached to the scalp record the combined activity of millions of neurons at the brain surface. The traces show distinctive patterns during sleep that demonstrate that it is not a consistent or uniform activity. In addition, sleep is different for everyone, varying in length, quality and depth (Rivkees 2003).

Cycles are also evident within sleep since characteristic cycles in brain wave patterns can be observed. There are times when the eyes make fast, flickering movements, in a type of sleep known as rapid eye movement (REM) sleep. This contrasts with a different kind of sleep called non-rapid eye movement (NREM) sleep. NREM sleep can be divided into different phases again. During a night's sleep there are discernible sleep patterns characterized by alternating periods of REM and NREM sleep.

The physiological processes that cause us to exhibit this sleep–wake cycle are still under investigation, as it is not clear precisely what makes us sleep and then wake. Because the sleep–wake cycle seems to reflect the dark–light cycle it seems logical that there is some connection between darkness and sleep, and light and wakefulness.

The clues to light and darkness being important for sleep come from studies with the pineal gland; this is a small gland in the brain which secretes a hormone called melatonin. The pineal gland is considered to be an important contributor to the biological timing system.

The SCN tracks fluctuations in light with the help of special light-sensitive cells in the retina. They send information about the duration and brightness of light to the pineal gland via a direct neural pathway, the retinohypothalamic tract (see Fig. 7.2) (Minors 1997, Wright 2002). In response to daylight the SCN emits signals that ultimately prevent melatonin being secreted from the pineal gland. After dark this inhibition lifts and melatonin secretion increases (Wright 2002). Increased melatonin levels correlate with sleep. At dawn, the pineal gland stops producing melatonin and wakefulness and alertness ensue (Morgan 1995, Minors 1997).

Pineal gland and melatonin secretion

Melatonin secretion exhibits a circadian rhythm with most melatonin being secreted during the night and little during the day. The rhythm of melatonin secretion appears to be due to two interacting influences, light and the endogenous rhythm of the pineal gland. Whilst melatonin secretion is influenced by light and dark cycles, the pattern of secretion also seems to result from internal body factors, since without any light or dark cues, melatonin secretion still follows a circadian rhythm (Morgan 1995). In humans, the pineal gland is not photosensitive and it relies on signals from the SCN, which promote secretion at night but not during daylight (Minors 1997).

Temperature rhythms are also influenced by melatonin secretion and it is possible that the effects of melatonin secretion on sleep inducement are indirect. The effects of melatonin on the sleep–wake cycle may be mediated via temperature regulation. Melatonin secretion at night may lead to thermoregulatory changes, heat loss mechanisms, which may promote sleep (Kräuchi & Wirz-Justice 2001, Kubota et al 2002). This may explain why bedtime behaviours, like warm baths, hot drinks and relaxation, which are all associated with vasodilation and heat loss, may increase sleepiness at night (Kräuchi & Wirz-Justice 2001).

Melatonin is a hormone synthesized from the amino acid tryptophan (Touitou 2001). As with other hormones, melatonin is secreted directly into the blood and can reach all cells in the body. It will only interact with cells that have melatonin receptors; these target cells are widely dispersed in the body. Melatonin has a variety of neuroendocrine roles (Reiter 1995), including influencing reproductive physiology (Pang et al 1998),

induction of sleep and contribution to circadian timing (Minors 1997), and influence on behaviour (Golumbek et al 1996), as well as antioxidant properties (Reiter 1995).

The secretion of melatonin changes throughout the human life cycle. Young children produce more melatonin (Touitou 2001) and this may contribute to explanations for their tendency to sleep longer than adults. Disruption of the rhythmicity of melatonin secretion and decreased circulating melatonin concentrations are linked to the increased incidence of sleep disorders in older people (Haimov et al 1994, Vitiello 1996). A number of different mechanisms that could account for the age-related decline in melatonin secretion and changes to the melatonin rhythm have been proposed, although there is still some debate about whether changes in melatonin rhythmicity are indeed a feature of ageing (Skene & Swaab 2003).

Seasonal timing is also thought to be regulated by the internal clock, suggesting that the pineal gland acts as a 'calendar' as well as playing a role in the biological timing system (Minors 1997). This yearly rhythm also has to be reset by some external zeitgeber, such as day length. Interestingly, progressive reduction in day length is correlated with seasonal affective disorder (SAD), a condition characterized by low mood or depression in winter when the days are shorter. It is ten times more common in northern latitudes (Wright 2002). Bright light therapy seems to resynchronize the secretion of melatonin and reverse the depressive symptoms (Morgan 1995, Partonen & Lonnqvist 1996).

Sleep centres

The brain controls sleep and responds to changes in the internal and external environment. An understanding of the structure and functions of the brain will illuminate the phenomenon of sleep and reveal the role of different brain components (see p. 91).

A number of components in the brain have been implicated in the initiation and maintenance of sleep. A 'sleep centre' is thought to exist in the reticular formation, a collection of nerve cells in the brain stem (see Fig. 7.3). The reticular formation is thought to include an activating system, which is known as the reticular activating system (Kayama 1995, Damasio 1999).

Sleep is associated with suppressed activity in the reticular formation, whilst arousal is associated with increased activity in the reticular formation. Nerve

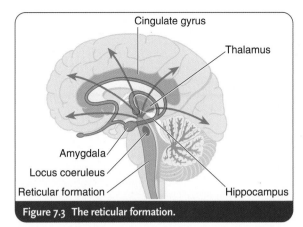

Figure 7.3 The reticular formation.

The arrows indicate projections from the reticular formation to the cerebral cortex. The locus coeruleus is part of the reticular formation. Activity in the thalamus, which is part of the limbic system, reflects the sleep–wake cycle. The cingulate gyrus, hippocampus and amygdala belong to the limbic system.

impulses go from the reticular formation to the thalamus, hypothalamus, cerebral cortex and other parts of the brain. When the activity in the reticular formation is inhibited, sleep occurs. The job of the reticular activating system is to keep the cerebral cortex in an awake state (Damasio 1999).

Some nuclei in the reticular formation seem to be particularly involved in sleep and wakefulness. There are three groups of neurons in the reticular formation that project to higher brain centres, and each uses a different neurotransmitter:

- neurons in the locus coeruleus (see Fig. 7.3) secrete noradrenaline, an excitatory neurotransmitter that activates the brain;
- neurons in the laterodorsal and pedunculopontine region secrete acetylcholine and are involved in REM sleep;
- neurons in the dorsal raphe secrete serotonin and their function remains unclear (Kayama 1995). The role of serotonergic neurons in sleep is complex; activity in different parts of the brain is associated with waking or sleeping depending on a range of factors including the receptor sub-type involved (Ursin 2002).

The thalamus has a key role in sleep; certain nuclei are responsible for projecting impulses to the cerebral cortex which result in the awake state or sleep state. During wakefulness the reticular formation generates a continuous volley of signals to the thalamus and cerebral cortex. It seems that nerve cells in both the reticular

formation and the thalamus fire these signals spontaneously. This activity in turn is modified by impulses carrying sensory information from the outside world to the brain (Damasio 1999). There are indications that the hypothalamus may also be part of the activating system, playing a significant role in waking (Lin 2000).

In addition to the reticular activating system whose activity is associated with wakefulness it is suggested there is an arousal inhibitory mechanism responsible for the transition from wakefulness to sleep. The mechanism is complex but involves a reduction in the activity reaching the thalamus and, ultimately, the cortex (Evans 2003).

Activity in the thalamus seems to reflect the sleep–wake cycle; during sleep there is less activity in the thalamus and it has a slow rhythmical pattern of theta and delta rhythms. Interestingly, slow, sleep-like activity in the thalamus seems to be a feature of patients with Parkinson's disease and this may account for the symptoms associated with the disease (Clayton 2000).

As indicated earlier, sleep comprises cycles, phases and stages. NREM, or orthodox sleep, is characterized by four stages: stages 1 and 2 represent light sleep and stages 3 and 4, deep sleep. REM sleep is characterized by rapid eye movements.

Non-rapid eye movement (NREM) sleep

Most sleep during the night is non-rapid eye movement (NREM) sleep or slow wave sleep. As many of the neurons are active at the same time, giving relatively large electrical signals, this activity was originally described as 'synchronized sleep'. Four stages can be described in the EEG during NREM sleep. The onset of sleep occurs in stage 1 as the person relaxes, mental activity becomes dream-like and brain waves are desynchronized. In stage 2 there is a progressive decline into delta waves, mental activity is characterized by wandering thoughts and the person is easily rousable. Stages 3 and 4 are deep sleep, brain waves are slow, muscles relax, temperature falls and there is a reduction in physiological reactivity to external stimuli (Moorcroft 1993, Duxbury 1994, Espie 2000).

NREM sleep seems to be a sort of restful state, associated with reduced heart rate and blood pressure, slow breathing and a lower basal metabolic rate. This kind of

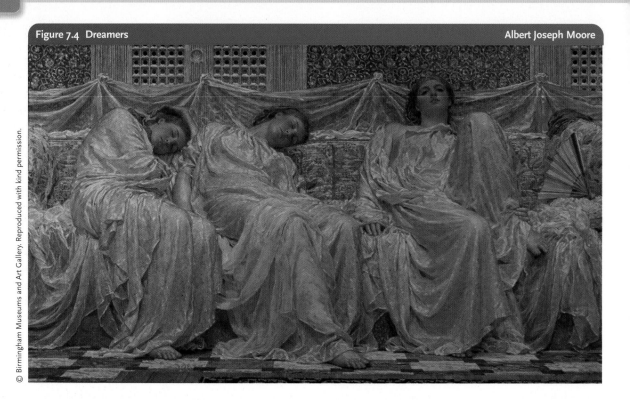

Figure 7.4 Dreamers   Albert Joseph Moore

sleep is sometimes known as 'dreamless sleep'. This cycle of sleep where the individual moves through the stages into deep sleep repeats four or five times a night. The amount of time spent in deepest sleep is particularly evident in the first part of the night (Rodéhn Fox 1999, Espie 2000).

Rapid eye movement sleep

REM sleep is sometimes called paradoxical sleep, the paradox being that the EEG pattern is like that of someone waking up, but the person is in a deep sleep. The brain wave activity reveals bursts of desynchronized beta waves. This type of sleep occurs 80–100 minutes after the onset of sleep and is then observed to occur at intervals, with each period of REM sleep lasting 5–30 minutes. The interval between each phase of REM sleep decreases during the night from about 90 minutes to 30 minutes towards morning. REM sleep occupies about 20% of the duration of a person's sleep (Moorcroft 1993, Rodéhn Fox 1999).

REM is associated with dreaming; if woken during this time then dreams are remembered (see Fig. 7.4). REM sleep is considered important in cognitive

wellbeing, information processing and memory formation (Duxbury 1994, Maquet et al 1996, Espie 2000). One theory is that dreaming may be the basis for processing memories (Greenfield 2000).

> ❛That night, sleeping deeply beneath her old quilted eiderdown, she had a sequence of dreams. They were mostly of the intensely realised but inconsequential kind that her father's friend had characterised as 'neural waste'.❜
>
> (Faulks 1999)

Functions of sleep

Sleep seems to be an essential component of health. Many theories about the purpose of sleep embrace the idea that sleep 'restores' us in some way (Duxbury 1994). The large 'pulses' of growth hormone released in sleep (Shalet 2000) are associated with protein synthesis and this is essential to make proteins such as collagen during wound healing. The hormones associated with reduced cell division are prevalent during wakefulness, whilst others involved with repair are active in sleep. This provides a mechanism to explain why 'rest is good for healing' (Hodgson 1991). Growth hormone secretion is especially increased in adolescents during sleep (Donovan 1988).

Sleep has also been considered as a type of behavioural adaptation to the environment. There are times when it might be safer to be asleep rather than awake; for example, predators might be more of a threat at night and the environment is more dangerous at night when you cannot see as well. Food may be more difficult to find at night so it also makes sense to sleep when food is less attainable (Moorcroft 1993).

Theories of the function of sleep also emphasize that sleep is essential for mental and emotional wellbeing and, as well as being implicated in memory formation, sleep is also thought to play a role in learning and mood modulation (Moorcroft 1993, Smith 1996).

> ❝ I'm drifting in and out of dreamless sleep
> Throwing all my memories in a ditch to keep. ❞
>
> (Bob Dylan 1997)

REM sleep is thought to be particularly important for normal brain function since selective deprivation of REM sleep is associated with increased anxiety, irritability and difficulty in concentration (Donovan 1988).

Sleep patterns throughout the human life cycle

Different patterns of sleep are evident during the various stages of the human life cycle. In children aged six years the mean time spent sleeping per day is about ten hours whilst young adults sleep for about seven hours (Moorcroft 1993, Morgan & Closs 1999). The proportion of REM sleep decreases with age. The higher proportion of REM sleep in newborns and infants suggests that REM sleep might be serving a function in brain development (Hobson 1989). As children get older they sleep more deeply whilst the total number of hours sleep decreases with age up to adulthood. Many changes in sleep occur during adolescence, reflecting changes in both physiology and behaviour. There

seems to be a dramatic decrease in the amount of sleep and the majority of teenagers are considered to be sleep deprived (Dahl & Lewin 2002).

Older people tend to fall asleep earlier and awaken earlier. Naps during the day contribute to a pattern of more sleep during the day and less sleep during the night compared to the younger adult. The number of awakenings and difficulty in returning to sleep after waking increases in older people. However, these are general trends and individual sleep patterns vary (Moorcroft 1993). Many possible causes have been suggested to account for the age-related changes in circadian rhythmicity and sleep patterns that occur. These include loss of nerve cells within the SCN, abnormalities in entrainment, insufficient time cues, and pineal gland dysfunction (Touitou 2001). Neurodegeneration within the SCN and lower melatonin levels are implicated in the pronounced disruption in circadian rhythmicity and sleep patterns demonstrated in Alzheimer's disease (Skene & Swaab 2003).

Sleep disorders

There are different types of sleep disorders relating to problems with the quantity, quality or timing of sleep. Insomnia or difficulty in sleeping is subjective and hence rather a vague term. Insomnia may be associated with existing psychological and medical disorders (Holbrook et al 2000).

Insomnia is the most common sleep disorder (Lichstein et al 2003) and is often viewed as a sign of an underlying disorder rather than a disorder itself (Harvey 2001). Insomnia can be viewed as a symptom of psychological disorders such as depression and anxiety, neurological disorders, medical disorders including arthritis, congestive heart failure, pain, and sleep disorders such as obstructive sleep apnoea and restless legs syndrome (Holbrook et al 2000, Harvey 2001). Alcohol, caffeine and a variety of drugs can also lead to insomnia (Holbrook et al 2000). The consequences of insomnia can be debilitating and may include stress, poor work performance, irritability and fatigue. Day time sleepiness is a feature of many sleep disorders and the risk of road traffic accidents is greater (Shapiro & Dement 1993). There is growing evidence of the link between sleep disorders and cardiovascular disease (Redeker 2002).

Another category of sleep disorders, the parasomnias, includes sleep terrors, sleepwalking, sleep talking, head banging, nightmares, and teeth grinding (Moorcroft 1993). Children are prone to many sleep disorders: 10–50% of children aged 3–5 years have nightmares (Shapiro & Dement 1993) whilst 3% have night terrors (Jaffa et al 1993). Nightmares occur in REM sleep and the child will remember them to some extent; night terrors, sleepwalking and sleep talking occur in deep sleep and are not usually remembered on waking in the morning (Jaffa et al 1993). Difficulties getting to sleep and remaining asleep are much more common, and can be due to a range of factors. A variety of strategies including behaviour modification may be employed to establish more appropriate bedtime routines and sleep patterns (Jaffa et al 1993).

Sleep disturbance and effects on mental health and wellbeing

Desynchronization between the sleep–wake cycle and the endogenous circadian pacemaker can have a profound effect on mood (Boivin et al 1997). Insomnia may precede the development of depression, anxiety and alcohol abuse (Harvey 2001). Sleep disturbances are present in nearly all psychopathological conditions. Apart from strong links with depression, sleep disturbance seems to be a characteristic of mania. The link between sleep loss and mania may be bidirectional, with sleep loss causing mania and mania causing sleep loss in a feedback loop (Wehr 1991).

Stress and life events are associated with sleep alterations and may relate to poor coping strategies. The preservation of normal social rhythms and sleep–wake rhythms during a stressful life event may protect individuals who are susceptible to depression (Riemann & Berger 1998). Individuals with a major depressive disorder often suffer with insomnia. Slow release melatonin seems to be successful in promoting sleep in these individuals in place of usual sleep medications (Dolberg et al 1998). The suggestion that there is a link between biological rhythm disturbances and major depressive disorders is longstanding, although most recent studies suggest that this is not related to circadian rhythm disturbance, but sleep disturbance particularly related to the timing of REM sleep (Armitage et al 1999). Dysregulation of ultradian (less than 24 hr) rhythms seems to be prevalent in depressed individuals with a breakdown in the organization of sleep EEG rhythms within and between the cerebral hemispheres (Armitage et al 1999).

Paradoxically, whilst sleep loss might be a predictor of depressive illness, sleep deprivation has been used successfully to ameliorate mood in depressed individuals. Thus it is apparent that stable sleep–wake rhythms are significant in maintaining and promoting mental health and wellbeing (Riemann & Berger 1998).

Comorbidity of insomnia with psychological disorders may also be significant in individuals with learning disabilities. Studies suggest that such individuals may suffer sleep–wake dysregulation characterized by spending more time in bed relative to sleep time and being prone to drowsiness, irritability and mood change during the day (Espie 2000). Disruption of the sleep–wake cycle could play an important role in the high prevalence of behavioural disorders in people with learning disabilities (Brylewski & Wiggs 1999).

Sleep promotion

Rest is an effective form of therapy; however, promoting sleep is challenging. The experience of rest and sleep is unique to different people and there are many factors that could promote rest for a particular individual (Narrow 2000). There are various strategies for sleep promotion including bedtime drinks, comfortable bedding, dimmed lighting, adequate ventilation, appropriate temperature, warm baths, bedtime rituals and sleep education programmes (Rodéhn Fox 1999, Floyd et al 2000). Sleep hygiene is the term given to managing sleep without using medication. Poor sleep hygiene refers to behavioural factors such as irregular sleep–wake cycles, frequent daytime napping and prolonged periods of time spent in bed trying to fall asleep (Riemann & Berger 1998). Characteristics of sleep hygiene would include a safe and comfortable place to sleep, adoption of pre-sleep rituals, regular getting up times and not sleeping too much (Moorcroft 1993). Additional strategies would be to avoid naps during the day and abstinence from alcohol, caffeine and other stimulants near to the start of sleep time.

In addition to the range of non-pharmacological strategies, there are various hypnotic drugs, mainly the benzodiazepines, used to promote sleep (Eisen et al 1993). A variety of dietary supplements such as valerian, tryptophan and melatonin are used by individuals to help them sleep despite the lack of data on their efficacy (Cauffield & Forbes 1999).

In summary, sleep is an essential component of health. It is a natural recurring state of unconsciousness, from which the individual can be aroused. A number of sleep centres in the brain are involved in controlling the sleep–wake cycle, together with melatonin from the pineal gland. The sleep–wake cycle is an important circadian rhythm; circadian rhythms are evident in a number of physiological processes and are crucial to maintaining homeostasis. Ill-health is associated with desynchronized circadian rhythms. There are two main types of sleep, REM sleep and NREM sleep, which have cycles throughout a night's sleep. Several functions are attributed to sleep, many of which are restorative.

Introducing the brain

The human brain is the most complex structure in the world, weighing about 1500 g and consisting of around 10^{11} neurons and about 10^{14} connections or synapses in total (McCrohan 2001). The human brain acts as an integrated whole with each nerve cell having connections with up to 20 000 other nerve cells, representing incredible complexity (Donovan 1988). The brain is made up of a number of components, which despite having key roles function together in an integrated way.

Cerebral hemispheres and cerebral cortex

The brain comprises the cerebrum made up of two halves, the left and right cerebral hemispheres connected by a bundle of fibres, the corpus callosum. The thin outer layer of the cerebral hemispheres is the cerebral cortex and constitutes the grey matter whilst the inner tissue is white matter. The cerebral cortex has a number of areas including the motor cortex and sensory cortex (see Fig. 7.5). The motor cortex controls voluntary movement and the somatosensory cortex receives and interprets information from receptors in the skin. Different parts of the body are mapped to particular areas in both the motor cortex and sensory cortex.

Each cerebral hemisphere has four lobes and a brief outline of their functions are given in Table 7.1.

Basal ganglia

The basal ganglia are collections of grey matter located deep within the white matter of cerebral hemispheres. Although the precise function of this group of nuclei is not completely understood, a major function is to control muscle activity. Motor impulses originating in the cerebral cortex are relayed through these ganglia. The basal ganglia play a key role in controlling various motor activities and they are also thought to have a role in timekeeping.

Thalamus

The thalamus acts like an old-fashioned telephone switchboard and is responsible for relaying almost all sensory information to the cerebral cortex. The thalamus receives impulses from the reticular formation in connection with the sleep–wake cycle. Impulses are projected from the thalamus to the cerebral cortex and contribute to waking.

Hypothalamus

The hypothalamus is composed of different areas with a range of roles. Although small in size, the hypothalamus is hugely significant in human brains. The hypothalamus controls eating behaviour and contains the 'satiety centre' (responsible for the feeling of fullness) and the 'hunger centre'. The hypothalamus is important in homeostasis since it is responsible for temperature regulation and fluid balance, and controls the autonomic nervous system. The hypothalamus integrates the mind and body. It is the physiological link to emotions and is associated with expressions of rage, sexual behaviour, pleasure and fear. The hypothalamus is an endocrine gland that produces a range of hormones, some of which control the activity of the anterior pituitary gland. It also influences sleep via the pineal gland and possibly via the activating system (Lin 2000).

Pineal gland

The pineal gland is shaped like a pine cone. Roughly the size of a pea, it is located in the roof of the third ventricle, which is deep within the brain. It secretes a hormone called melatonin which has many roles including the initiation of sleep (see also p. 86).

Limbic system

The limbic system is a collection of components rather than a specific part; it is sometimes known as the emotional brain. It is a complex system of nerve pathways

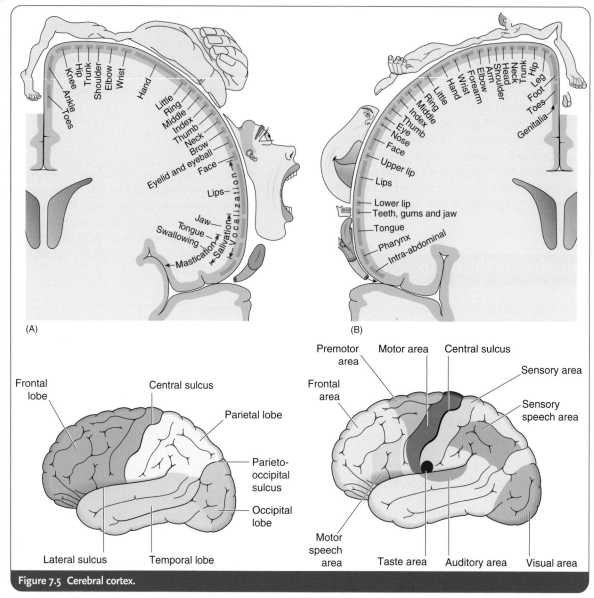

Figure 7.5 Cerebral cortex.

The lobes and functional areas of the cerebral cortex. Parts of the body are mapped onto areas of the sensory and motor cortex. (A) Motor cortex. (B) Sensory cortex. (Reproduced with kind permission from Waugh & Grant 2001.)

and contains collections of grey matter of the cerebral cortex (see Fig. 7.3). The limbic system is involved with feeding behaviour, aggression, expression of emotion and the autonomic, behavioural and hormonal aspects of sexual response. Olfaction plays a role in triggering these types of behaviour. The amygdala, part of the limbic system, is associated with aggression, food and water intake. The hippocampus, another component, is involved in changing short-term memory to long-term memory.

Brain stem

The brain stem consists of the midbrain, pons varolli and medulla oblongata. The midbrain controls cranial reflex activities such as blinking, ducking the head to visual stimuli and the pupillary reflex. It is responsible for the integration of incoming messages and is connected with visual and auditory perception. The pons is a 'bridge' between the higher brain and spinal cord, and has centres associated with the control of breathing.

breathing, heart activity and blood pressure control.

Reticular formation

This is a thick cluster of neurons within the brain stem and is the principal area involved in the regulation of attention and arousal. The reticular activating system is part of the reticular formation and is involved in states of alertness and waking.

Cerebellum

The cerebellum has three key functions, which include controlling skeletal muscle activity, regulating muscle tone and controlling balance. It acts as a filter to smooth and coordinate muscular activity in skilled voluntary muscle movements.

This overview of the components that make up the brain and their key functions is just a very small step towards beginning to understand the brain! Discovering the relationship of the physical entity of the brain to concepts such as the mind, emotions and consciousness will be a fascinating challenge.

Table 7.1 Functional roles of lobes in the cerebrum

Lobe	Summary of key roles
Frontal	**Motor functions**: Primary and secondary motor areas within the frontal lobe play a key role in controlling voluntary skeletal muscle movements. Broca's area is responsible for articulating words, it coordinates complex muscular actions of mouth, tongue and larynx in speech. Usually found in left hemisphere. **Integrative functions**: Control of emotional expressions, moral and ethical behaviour. Higher intellectual functions including concentrating, planning, problem solving and judgement. Creativity. Personality.
Parietal	**Sensory functions**: Receives and processes information from receptors in the skin, joints, muscles and organs. Responsible for sensations of touch, temperature, pressure and pain. **Integrative functions**: Contributes to the understanding of speech and choosing words to express thoughts and feelings.
Temporal	**Sensory functions**: Roles in hearing, balance and sense of smell. **Integrative functions**: Understanding speech. Plays a role in emotions and memory.
Occipital	**Sensory functions**: Contains the visual cortex and is responsible for vision. **Integrative functions**: Making visual images meaningful by combining visual images with other sensory experiences.

A small area of the pons is called the locus coeruleus. This area is associated with anxiety and mood disorders. Neurons from here project to higher centres and are also involved in the reticular activating system. The medulla contains vital centres for the control of

References

Armitage R, Hoffman R F, Rush A J 1999 Biological rhythm disturbance in depression: temporal coherence of ultradian sleep EEG rhythms. Psychological Medicine 29(6):1435–1448

Baxendale S, Clancy J, McVicar A 1997 Clinical implications of circadian rhythmicity for nurses and patients. British Journal of Nursing 6(6):303–309

Boivin D B, Czeisler C A, Dijk D-J et al 1997 Complex interaction of the sleep–wake cycle and circadian phase modulates mood in healthy subjects. Archives of General Psychiatry 54(2):145–152

Brylewski J, Wiggs L 1999 Sleep problems and daytime challenging behaviour in a community-based sample of adults with intellectual disability. Journal of Intellectual Disability Research 43:504–512

Cauffield J S, Forbes H J M 1999 Dietary supplements used in the treatment of depression, anxiety and sleep disorders. Lippincott's Primary Care Practice 3(3):290–304

Clancy J, McVicar A 1994a Circadian rhythms 1: physiology. British Journal of Nursing 3(13):657–661

Clancy J, McVicar A 1994b Circadian rhythms 2: shiftwork and health. British Journal of Nursing 3(14):712–717

Clayton J 2000 Caught napping. New Scientist 165(2227):42–45

Dahl R E, Lewin D S 2002 Pathways to adolescent health sleep regulation and behaviour. Journal of Adolescent Health 31(6) Supplement 1:175–184

Damasio A 1997 The feeling of what happens. Heinemann, London

Dijk D-J 1996 Internal rhythms in humans. Seminars in Cell & Developmental Biology 7:831–836

Dolberg O, Hirschmann S, Grunhaus L 1998 Melatonin for the treatment of sleep disturbances in major depressive disorder. American Journal of Psychiatry 155(8):1119–1121

Donovan B T 1988 Humors, hormones and the mind. Macmillan Press, London

Duxbury J 1994 Understanding the nature of sleep. Nursing Standard 9(9):25–28

Dylan B 1997 Million miles. Time out of mind. Columbia

Eisen J, MacFarlane J, Shapiro C M 1997 Psychotropic drugs and sleep. In: Shapiro C M (ed) ABC of sleep disorders. BMJ Publishing Group, London, p 66–69

Espie C A 2000 Sleep and disorders of sleep in people with mental retardation. Current Opinion in Psychiatry 13(5):507–511

Evans B M 2003 Sleep, consciousness and the spontaneous and evoked electrical activity of the brain. Is there a cortical integrating mechanism? Clinical Neurophysiology 33(1):1–10

Faulks S 1997 Charlotte Gray. Vintage, London, p 479

Floyd J A, Falahee M L, Fhobir R H 2000 Creation and analysis of a computerised database of interventions to facilitate adult sleep. Nursing Research 49(4):236–241

Greenfield S 2000 The private life of the brain. Penguin, London

Golombek D A, Pévet P, Cardinali D P 1996 Melatonin effects on behaviour: possible mediation by the central GABAergic system. Neuroscience and Biobehavioral Reviews 20(3):403–412

Haimov I, Laudon M, Zisapel N et al 1994 Sleep disorders and melatonin rhythms in elderly people. British Medical Journal 309(6948): 167

Harvey A G 2001 Insomnia: symptom or diagnosis. Clinical Psychology Review 21(7):1037–1059

Hobson J A 1989 Sleep. Scientific American Library, New York

Hodgson L 1991 Why do we need sleep? Relating theory to nursing practice. Journal of Advanced Nursing 16:1503–1510

Holbrook A M, Crowther R, Lotter A et al 2000 The diagnosis and management of insomnia in clinical practice: a practical evidence-based approach. Canadian Medical Association Journal 162(2):210–216

Jaffa T, Scott S, Hendriks J, Shapiro C M 1993 Sleep disorders in children. In: Shapiro C M (ed) ABC of sleep disorders. BMJ Publishing Group, London, p 41–44

Kayama Y 1995 Ascending reticular activating system revisited: functional roles of cholinergic and monoaminergic projections from the brain stem. Electroencephalography and Clinical Neurophysiology 97(4):S44

Kräuchi K, Wirz-Justice A 2001 Circadian clues to sleep onset mechanisms. Neuropsychopharmacology 25(S5):S92–96

Kubota T, Uchiyama M, Suzuki H et al 2002 Effects of bright light on saliva melatonin, core body temperature and sleep propensity rhythms in human subjects. Neuroscience 42:115–122

Lichstein K L, Durrence H H, Taylor D J et al 2003 Quantitative criteria for insomnia. Behaviour Research and Therapy 41(4):427–445

Lin J S 2000 Brain structures and mechanisms involved in the control of cortical activation and wakefulness, with emphasis on the posterior hypothalamus and histaminergic neurons. Sleep Medicine Reviews 4(5):471–503

Maquet P, Peters J M, Aerts J et al 1996 Functional neuro-anatomy of human rapid-eye movement sleep and dreaming. Nature 383(6596):163–166

Martensen R L 1995 The somnolence of sleep research. Journal of the American Medical Association 274(20):1643

McCaughrean G 1994 Stories from the Ballet. Orchard Books, London, p 106

McCrohan C 2001 Making the connection. Biological Sciences Review 13(3):10–13

McCrone J 1997 When a second lasts forever. New Scientist 156(2106):52–56

Minors D 1997 Melatonin: hormone of darkness. Biological Sciences Review 10(1):39–41

Morgan E 1995 Measuring time with a biological clock. Biological Sciences Review 7(4):2–5

Morgan K, Closs S J 1999 Sleep management in nursing practice. Churchill Livingstone, Edinburgh

Moorcroft W H 1993 Sleep, dreaming, and sleep disorders, 2nd edn. University Press of America, Maryland

Narrow B W 2000 Rest is.... American Journal of Nursing 100(10):96SS–96YY

Oswald I 1966 Sleep. Penguin Books, Harmondsworth

Pang S F, Li L, Ayre E A et al 1998 Neuroendocrinology of melatonin in reproduction: recent developments. Journal of Chemical Neuroanatomy 14(3–4):157–166

Partonen T, Lonnqvist J 1996 Prevention of winter seasonal affective disorder by bright-light treatment. Psychological Medicine 26(5):1075–1080

Redeker N S 2002 Foreword: Sleep and cardiovascular disease. Journal of Cardiovascular Nursing 17(1):v–ix

Reiter R J 1995 Functional pleiotropy of the neurohormone melatonin: antioxidant protection and neuroendocrine regulation. Frontiers in Neuroendocrinology 16(4):383–415

Riemann D, Berger M 1998 Sleep disorders and mental disorders. Current Opinion in Psychiatry 11(3):327–331

Rivkees S A 2003 Time to wake-up to the individual variation in sleep needs. Journal of Clinical Endocrinology and Metabolism 88(1):24–25

Rodéhn Fox M 1999 The importance of sleep. Nursing Standard 13(24):44–47

Shalet S 2000 Growth hormone: the elixir of youth? Biological Sciences Review 12(4):26–28

Shapiro C M, Dement W C 1993 Impact and epidemiology of sleep disorders. In: Shapiro C M (ed) ABC of sleep disorders. BMJ Publishing Group, London, p 1–4

Skene D J, Swaab D F 2003 Melatonin rhythmicity: effect of age and Alzheimer's disease. Experimental Gerontology 38:199–206

Smith C 1996 Sleep states, memory processes and synaptic plasticity. Behavioral Brain Research 78(1):49–56

Thompson D 1992 The time of onset of heart attacks. Nursing Standard 6(20):33–34

Touitou Y 2001 Human aging and melatonin. Clinical relevance. Experimental Gerontology 36:1083–1100

Ursin R 2002 Serotonin and sleep. Sleep Medicine Review 6(1):55–67

Vitiello M V 1996 Sleep disorders and aging. Current Opinion in Psychiatry 9(4):284–289

Waterhouse J, Minors D 1993 Circadian rhythms. In: Shapiro C M (ed) ABC of sleep disorders. BMJ Publishing Group, London, p 30–33

Waugh A, Grant A 2001 Ross and Wilson: Anatomy and physiology in health and illness. Churchill Livingstone, Edinburgh

Wehr T A 1991 Sleep loss as a possible mediator of diverse causes of trauma. British Journal of Psychiatry 159:576–578

Weiner J 1999 Time, love, memory. Faber and Faber, London

Wright K 2002 Times of our lives. Scientific American 287(3):41–47

Young M W 2000 The tick-tock of the biological clock. Scientific American 282(3):46–53

8

PAIN

❝The relief of pain and suffering has been a continuing human endeavour since the dawn of recorded history. Yet despite centuries of observation and study, we are only beginning to understand the subtleties and complexities of pain.❞

(Melzack 1973)

Pain is a phenomenon that all of us can describe from first-hand experience, yet trying to understand the puzzle of pain is difficult. Pain is complex; it is much more than a physiological sensation. It is an unpleasant experience that has both physiological and psychological attributes shaped by the sociocultural context. Because a person's experience of pain is unique to them, it is often difficult to understand the precise nature of their experience. 'Pain is whatever the experiencing person says it is, existing whenever the experiencing person says it does' (McCaffery 1968, cited in McCaffery & Pasero 1999, p. 17).

There are different types of pain; some pain is protective and acts as an early warning to alert the individual that tissue damage is or about to occur. The pain that is felt following an injury helps to prevent further damage during healing and repair (Woolf 1995). Pain can be experienced when there is no evidence of tissue damage and phantom pains can be felt in a missing limb (Haigh & Blake 2001). Any definition of pain has to encompass all these different manifestations. The International Association for the Study of Pain (IASP) (1979) defines pain as 'an unpleasant sensory and emotional experience associated with actual or potential tissue damage or described in terms of such damage' (cited by Merskey 1994, p. 904). This definition of pain acknowledges that pain is an experience not just a sensation – it suggests that pain has different dimensions, sensory and emotional, and acknowledges that pain cannot always be linked to actual tissue damage.

The experience of pain is not a simple straightforward response to an unpleasant sensation. The perception and response to pain are dependent on many factors including the individual's emotional state, memories, muscle movement, other sensory inputs and the cultural, environmental and socio-economic context. For example, the sensation of warm water in a bath can reduce pain whilst feeling unhappy or moving an injured limb might make the pain worse.

Pain is a multidimensional experience with physical, psychological, social, cultural and spiritual components. Pain also has a cognitive component – the individual thinks about pain, its meaning, significance and impact on wellbeing (Casey 1996).

❝Pain is not just a sensation but, like hunger and thirst, is an awareness of an action plan to be rid of it.❞

(Wall 1999, epilogue)

Components in the pain pathway

All sensations including pain depend on nerve connections between the periphery and the central nervous system. When nerve impulses reach the sensory cortex in the brain, the sensation is localized to a particular body part. All sensory information follows the same kind of neural pathway. Whilst the processing of pain information is more complex, the flow of information follows a similar pattern. Receptors respond to pain stimuli and pain information is carried by sensory neurons to the spinal cord, where pain information is processed and continues to the brain via ascending tracts in the spinal cord (Monafo 1995). Each of these steps in the neural mechanisms involved in the pain experience will be addressed in turn.

Pain stimuli

Stimuli that elicit pain are called noxious stimuli and include physical and chemical stimuli. Physical stimuli include intense or noxious thermal and mechanical stimuli. Physical stimuli such as a burn or a physical blow produce immediate pain, but chemicals released as a result of tissue damage can then also cause further pain (McHugh & McHugh 2000). Various chemicals, including hydrogen ions, potassium ions, prostaglandins, histamine, bradykinin and serotonin, released as a result of tissue damage will stimulate nociceptors (pain receptors) which respond to noxious chemicals (Cross 1994).

Types of tissue damage that cause pain include a deficiency of blood (ischaemia) and subsequent deficiency of oxygen (hypoxia); ulceration, infection, nerve damage and inflammation. In all cases pain-stimulating chemicals will accumulate and trigger the cycle of events that cause pain.

Nociceptors

Nociceptors are bare nerve endings found next to mast cells and small blood vessels, the three components function together to respond to pain (McHugh & McHugh 2000). They are found in the skin, muscle, joint capsules, visceral organs and arterial walls (Barasi 1991).

There appear to be two types of nociceptor, with different roles to play in pain transmission. The high threshold mechanoceptor responds to intense mechanical stimuli and the polymodal nociceptor responds to noxious mechanical, thermal and chemical stimuli (Barasi 1991, Cross 1994, McHugh & McHugh 2000).

Nociception

Nociception is the term that describes the events that occur in nociceptors, which convert pain stimuli into nerve impulses. This conversion of noxious stimuli into nerve impulses is not yet clearly understood, but begins when noxious stimuli provoke an inflammatory response causing mast cells to release chemical mediators such as histamine. Cell injury also leads to the release of arachidonic acid from the cell membrane, stimulating the synthesis of prostaglandins, thromboxanes and leukotrienes. Bradykinin is also produced as a result of tissue injury (Barasi 1991, Monafo 1995). All these chemical mediators contribute to the generation of pain stimuli in complex ways (McHugh & McHugh 2000).

Nociceptor endings secrete a range of neuropeptides including substance P and the amino acid glutamate in response to histamine. These neurochemicals further stimulate the nociceptors and mast cells. This interplay and escalation of various chemicals act on the nociceptor and ultimately leads to the opening of ion channels

and the generation of action potentials in the nerve fibres leading off from the nociceptors (McHugh & McHugh 2000). The prolonged release of histamine and substance P helps to explain why pain is still experienced after the noxious stimulus has been removed.

Chemicals such as bradykinin, prostaglandins and leukotrienes released following injury can sensitize nociceptors, making stimuli that are not normally painful cause pain; this is experienced as tenderness and pain beyond the initial injury site. Sensitization describes the phenomenon of neurons becoming more sensitive to pain. Sensitized neurons may respond to weaker stimuli, respond more intensely and may fire off pain impulses spontaneously (Cross 1994). This sensitization of nociceptors leads to tenderness described as hyperalgaesia (Monafo 1995, Woolf 1995, McHugh & McHugh 2000).

The sensitization of nociceptors also helps to explain postoperative pain. The initial surgical incision is of short duration, but the pain following surgery may last for hours and days. This is because sensitized nociceptors continue to send nerve impulses without being stimulated by pain stimuli. The nociceptors have become sensitized by the chemicals released following the injury in the inflammatory response. The stimulation of nociceptors has moved from mechanical to chemical stimuli postoperatively. The reduced threshold of sensitized nociceptors may allow them to respond to non-pain stimuli such as touch and gentle heat (Treede 1995).

Non-steroidal anti-inflammatory drugs (NSAIDs) such as aspirin and ibuprofen help to reduce pain because they prevent the formation of prostaglandins. Since prostaglandins play a role in sensitization, without them the nociceptors are less likely to become sensitized and, therefore, fewer pain impulses will be transmitted (Cross 1994, Woolf 1995).

Transmission of pain impulses to the spinal cord

There are two types of fibres for conducting pain nerve impulses; they are the relatively small A-delta fibres and the even smaller C fibres. These sensory fibres carry the pain information from the nociceptors to the dorsal horn in the spinal cord (p. 105) (Monafo 1995).

Of the two types, A-delta fibres have a slightly larger diameter and are myelinated; both these attributes enable this type of fibre to carry pain impulses more quickly. They carry nerve impulses at a speed of about six to eight metres per second (Monafo 1995) and are sometimes referred to as fast fibres. These fibres connect to the high threshold mechanoreceptors. The C fibres are smaller diameter unmyelinated fibres, which therefore have a slower conduction velocity of about one metre per second. These fibres are often referred to as slow fibres and they connect to the polymodal receptor (Barasi 1991).

Sometimes a distinction between 'first' and 'second' pain is made. The first pain is the pricking or sharp pain associated with A-delta fibres and the second or burning, dull aching, poorly localized pain is associated with C fibres (Jackson 1995, McHugh & McHugh 2000). However, there is some debate about the physiological basis of these classifications (Barasi 1991). The second pain persists after the acute pain stimulus has ceased and is associated with affective–motivational aspects of pain (Cross 1994).

There are other types of sensory nerve fibres not associated with carrying pain information, including A-beta fibres. These fibres are thicker than both types of pain fibres and therefore conduct impulses more quickly. They are often referred to as large diameter afferent fibres (Barasi 1991).

Spinal cord processing

A-delta and C fibres carry pain information to the dorsal horn of the spinal cord. The grey matter in the spinal cord is highly organized into a number of layers, called lamina. Within the spinal cord, each afferent fibre is likely to synapse with many interneurons (small linking neurons) located in different regions (or laminae) of the spinal cord. Afferent fibres carrying pain information tend to terminate and synapse with interneurons in the superficial laminae of the dorsal horn (Barasi 1991). The site where the majority of C and A-delta fibres terminate and where pain is modulated in the spinal cord is called the substantia gelatinosa (Dickenson 1995). In the dorsal horn, the C fibres and A-delta fibres form synapses with neurons that cross over to the opposite side of the spinal cord and carry impulses up towards the brain.

Transmission of noxious information to the brain

Pain information reaches the brain via a number of ascending tracts; these are columns of sensory neurons carrying nerve impulses to the brain. An important spinal cord pathway for signalling pain stimuli is the lateral spinothalamic tract (Barasi 1991, Cross 1994). Fibres in this tract carry pain information from the

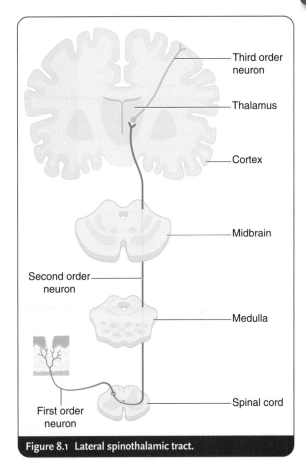

Figure 8.1 Lateral spinothalamic tract.

Three sensory neurons carry pain information to the brain in this pathway.

spinal cord to the thalamus in the brain. In the thalamus, another neuron then relays the noxious information to the cerebral cortex. In this pain pathway, three sensory neurons have carried noxious input from the periphery to the brain. The first order neuron carries nerve impulses from the nociceptor and synapses in the dorsal horn with the second order neuron. This neuron crosses over to the other side of the spinal cord and forms part of the spinothalamic tract which terminates in the thalamus. A third-order neuron conducts the pain information from the thalamus to the sensory cortex (see Fig. 8.1).

Fibres from the thalamus also project into the limbic system, basal ganglia and hypothalamus. The projection of fibres carrying pain information to the hypothalamus explains the autonomic changes associated with pain. The physiological responses to pain are mediated by the sympathetic nervous system and include pallor, sweating, nausea, increased heart rate, dilated pupils, increased blood pressure and an increased respiratory rate (O'Hara 1996).

Fibres from the thalamus project to many sites in the brain stem and this could account for the multiple components of pain, including sensory, arousal and autonomic aspects (Price 1995). Fibres from the thalamus may also project to the frontal lobes, which are important for the behavioural or affective component of pain (Monafo 1995). Many fibres from the thalamus project into the limbic system where the emotional aspects of pain and responses associated with it, such as anxiety and fear, are generated. The amygdala is thought to play an important role in the affective, emotional, behavioural and autonomic responses to pain (Bernard & Besson 1990).

The anterior cingulate cortex appears to play a role in integrating information about pain perception. Pain alerts the individual to tissue damage, helps to signify how serious the danger might be and then promotes learning so that the danger is remembered and avoided in the future. The anterior cingulate cortex seems to collate all these fragments of information together (Motluk 1999) and is involved in the perception of suffering and emotional response (Cross 1994). There are numerous opioid receptors in this region that may be influential in modulating the pain experience (Cross 1994, Derbyshire 2002).

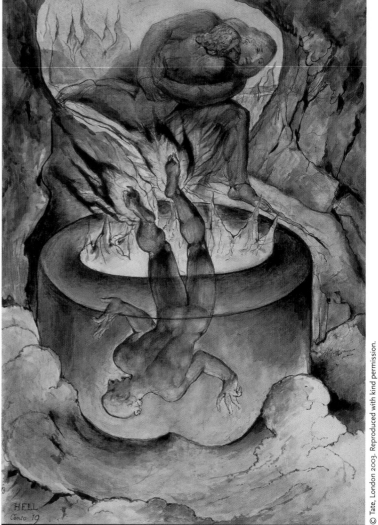

Figure 8.2 The Simoniac Pope 1824–1827   **William Blake**

Gate control theory of pain

Our understanding and theories about pain perception and response have evolved through many stages (see Fig. 8.2). Pain was originally thought to be due to evil spirits and demons rather than any injury. When the source of pain was understood to be located within the body, the Egyptians, Assyrians and Babylonians thought the heart rather than the brain was the organ that experienced pain (Astley 1990).

In 1644, Descartes developed theories on bodily sensations and outlined a mechanism of pain. He proposed that nerve threads lead directly from the skin to the brain. He envisaged that, rather like pulling a rope at the bottom of a tower will ring a bell attached at the top, pain in the foot could send particles to the brain where the pain would be felt. Given this rudimentary explanation of pain, Descartes surprisingly had innovative ideas about phantom pain and recognized that the pain felt was real (Rey 1995).

Centuries later, Melzack and Wall (1965) developed the gate control theory of pain which explains how pain can be modulated in the spinal cord. This theory embraces the interaction of the physiological, psychological and sociocultural factors that lead to pain perception and response. They proposed the concept of a gating mechanism in the dorsal horn of the spinal cord

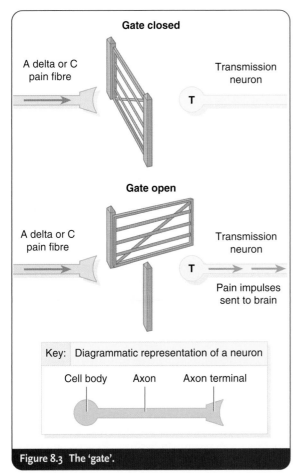

Figure 8.3 The 'gate'.

The pain fibre synapses with the transmission neuron in the dorsal horn of the spinal cord. These diagrams illustrate the concept of the 'gate' that controls the flow of pain information to the brain. The arrows represent pain impulses.

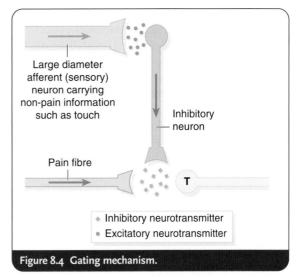

Figure 8.4 Gating mechanism.

The gating mechanism in the spinal cord relies on a small inhibitory neuron which when active suppresses the flow of pain information to the brain. The arrows represent nerve impulses.

through which pain information had to pass on its way to the brain. The opening and closing of the gate to pain information can be influenced by a number of different factors.

Nerve impulses from nociceptors and their sensory fibres (A-delta or C fibres) arrive in the dorsal horn of the spinal cord in the substantia gelatinosa. Here they synapse with the second-order neurons, which are often referred to as transmission (T) neurons. Axons from the T neurons project to the brain via a number of the pain pathways, including the lateral spinothalamic tract (see Fig. 8.1).

When information flows from A-delta or C pain fibres across the synapse to the T neuron via the secretion of excitatory neurotransmitters, the gate is said to be 'open' (see Fig. 8.3). The closing of the gate is achieved when the T neurons are inhibited by chemical neurotransmitters.

The excitatory neurotransmitters secreted by the A-delta or C pain fibres are glutamate and substance P. The relative importance of these two neurotransmitters is unclear (McHugh & McHugh 2000).

At the synapse between the pain fibres (A-delta or C fibres) and the T neuron are small interneurons (see Fig. 8.4). The T neurons are influenced by the activity of these small inhibitory interneurons in the substantia gelatinosa. As their name suggests when activated, these inhibitory neurons suppress the flow of pain information to the brain by inhibiting the T neurons.

Large diameter sensory neurons carrying sensory information such as touch, pressure and temperature, but not pain, synapse with the interneuron. Impulses arriving at the synapse along these sensory neurons excite the interneuron. The neurotransmitters secreted from these non-pain, large diameter fibres are excitatory amino acids and glutamate in particular (McHugh & McHugh 2000). Once excited, the inhibitory inter-neurons transmit nerve impulses that cause inhibitory neurotransmitters to be secreted at the synapse with the T neuron. Inhibition of the T neuron suppresses the flow of pain information towards the brain (see Fig. 8.4).

The large diameter sensory (or afferent) neurons are myelinated, which means that they transmit nerve impulses more quickly than the pain fibres. Stimulation of these large diameter fibres suppresses the transmission of impulses from the small diameter pain fibres to the T neuron.

In summary, activity in the large diameter fibres tends to close the gate whilst activity in the smaller pain fibres tends to facilitate transmission and opens the gate. The theory also suggests that it is the relative amount of activity in the two functionally distinct fibres which determines the pain intensity. As the activity in large diameter fibres increases less pain is perceived, whilst more activity in the small diameter pain fibres means more pain is felt (Barasi 1991).

This phenomenon helps to explain why rubbing your toe after hurting it helps to relieve the pain. Other types of sensory information, massage, gentle heat or cold can also help to relieve pain (Barasi 1991). Not only can other types of sensory inputs from the periphery modulate pain, but so can information that descends from the brain.

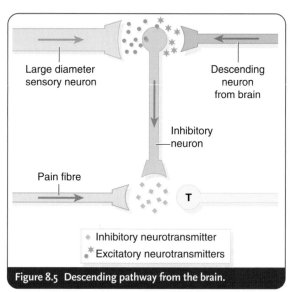

Figure 8.5 Descending pathway from the brain.

Descending pathways can also suppress the flow of pain information by stimulating the inhibitory neuron.

Descending pathways modulate the flow of pain information

The gate theory also proposes that information flowing down descending inhibitory pathways from higher brain centres closes the 'gate'. The descending pain-control pathways are the basis for psychological factors that modulate pain. The fibres of the descending pathways originate in the reticular formation (Cross 1994) in the periaqueductal grey matter (PAGM) and raphe nuclei (Barasi 1991, O'Hara 1996).

The descending neurons which arise in the brain, synapse with the inhibitory interneurons in the substantia gelatinosa. As nerve impulses transmitted by descending neurons arrive at the synapse, they cause neurotransmitters such as serotonin and noradrenaline to be secreted (Barasi 1991). These neurotransmitters then excite the inhibitory neuron, which suppresses pain transmission in the T neuron to the brain (see Fig. 8.5).

The inhibitory neuron secretes natural opioids (enkephalins, dynorphins and endorphins) and these peptides inhibit the T neuron. These are the body's natural 'pain killers' and this mechanism is sometimes called the natural analgesic system. The natural opioids, enkephalins in particular, inhibit the flow of pain information in two ways: they block the release of substance P (the neurotransmitter secreted by pain fibres) and they block receptors for substance P on the T neuron.

The inhibitory interneuron can be excited either by the descending pathway or by sensory information arriving at the synapse in large diameter sensory fibres. In both cases the T neuron will be inhibited by the natural opioids secreted from the inhibitory neuron and the flow of pain information to the brain will be suppressed (Barasi 1991).

The complexity of pain is highlighted by the role of descending pathways. Early studies on these pathways related to phenomena associated with acute stimuli whereas more recent studies have focused on chronic pain conditions. It now seems that the descending modulation of pain has two dimensions, inhibition and facilitation. The balance and timing between facilitation and inhibition is crucial and shifts in this balance may contribute to chronic pain conditions (Ren & Dubner 2002).

Acute pain and chronic pain

Traditionally, pain that has a recent onset and is only short-lived is acute pain, whilst persistent pain is described as chronic pain. Acute pain encompasses pain of different magnitudes and durations, but does not persist beyond three months (Treede 1995). Acute pain commonly refers to pain that is sudden in onset and severe in nature, although the pain intensity can vary from mild to severe (O'Hara 1996). Acute pain is associated with surgery, medical illness such as myocardial infarction and sickle cell crisis, and musculoskeletal pain like rheumatoid arthritis, cancer, trauma, burns and labour pain (McQuay & Moore 1998).

Chronic pain is traditionally defined as pain that lasts for more than three months (Merskey 1986). However, chronic pain is a syndrome, it is not just persistent acute pain. Acute pain can become chronic pain rapidly (Carr & Goudas 1999). Acute pain is the body's alarm system; it signals that something is wrong or that you are in danger of injury. However, chronic pain serves no such purpose and can cause endless suffering (Breen 2002).

Even after a brief acute pain, changes may occur within the spinal cord in the first few hours resulting in chronic pain (Dickenson 1995). This illustrates the plasticity of the nervous system which can be moulded, remodelled or changed by experiences such as pain. Acute pain may be considered as the first phase of pain. The intensity, duration, quality and meaning of the pain for the individual and the variety of factors influencing the initial pain experience are all instrumental in shaping how the pain experience unfolds, including the possible progression to chronic pain (Carr & Goudas 1999).

Sensitization

Sensitization leads to pain hypersensitivity. As described earlier, peripheral sensitization occurs due to the release of chemical mediators such as prostaglandins and this leads to pain hypersensitivity in a localized area around the injured site (Woolf 1995). This peripheral sensitization causes the pain felt when a grazed knee is put in a warm bath – the usually pleasant sensation of warm water on the skin has become painful.

Central sensitization occurs in spinal neurons. Neurons that become used to carrying pain information can become sensitized, that is, the neurons conducting pain information undergo changes in sensitivity so that ordinary sensory information such as pressure on an injured foot becomes transformed into pain information. This helps to explain why the pain someone feels may be out of proportion to the tissue damage (Youngson 1992).

Central sensitization is implicated in postoperative pain. There is evidence that pre-emptive management of pain can reduce postoperative pain (Youngson 1992). The use of local anaesthesia at the incision site prior to surgery is thought to stop nerve impulses being transmitted to the spinal cord and brain, and heightened sensitivity can be avoided (Roberge & McEwen 1998). Pre-emptive analgesia prevents central sensitization from occurring and therefore may reduce postoperative pain (Woolf 1995).

Chemicals released within the spinal cord mediate the transmission of pain signals. N-methyl-D-aspartate (NMDA) receptors are implicated in the mechanism that causes spinal cord neurons to become hypersensitive. Sensitization can result in non-painful stimuli causing pain and may lead to pain from a minor injury developing into severe pain. NMDA receptors are activated by the neurotransmitter glutamate (see p. 60). Activation of these receptors leads to plasticity within the spinal cord (Liu et al 1997); the neurons become more sensitive to incoming signals, the synapses behaving as though they have gained strength.

The phenomenon of sensitization illustrates that pain is an active process rather than just a relay of noxious information to the brain. Sensitization occurring in both the periphery and spinal cord reflects neuronal plasticity and leads to pain hypersensitivity (Woolf & Salter 2000).

Neuropathic pain

Neuropathic pain is pain that follows injury to the peripheral or central nervous system itself rather than the pain described so far, which is nociceptive pain. Nociceptive pain results from activation of nociceptors in somatic or visceral tissues and the transmission of nerve impulses through an intact nervous system. Somatic pain arises from injury of the skin, mucosa, muscle and bone. Visceral pain is caused by stimulation of nociceptors in internal organs due to tissue damage such as distension, inflammation, obstruction, infection and ischaemia in organs such as the stomach, kidney, gall bladder, intestines and bladder (Al-Chaer & Traub 2002).

Neuropathic pain is a complex and chronic pain with the potential to be severe and persistent (Woolf 1995). Individuals with neuropathic pain describe pain as burning, stabbing and shooting. Nerve injuries may be due to trauma or to diseases such as diabetes and AIDS or following herpes infections. Phantom limb pain is also neuropathic pain (Lynch 2001). There are a variety of painful symptoms associated with neuropathic pain, including unusual sensations such as pins and needles, numbness, tingling, cramp and feelings of tightness. Each person's experience of neuropathic pain is unique. Both peripheral sensitization and central sensitization contribute to the hypersensitivity experienced in neuropathic pain (Wilson 2002).

Biological basis of pain management

The control of pain is inevitably complex. It is crucial to control early pain since this can influence the subsequent pain experience (Carr & Goudas 1999). The goal of pain management is to achieve optimal comfort, promote function and minimize side effects (Lynch 2001). Successful pain management includes removing or managing the cause of pain. Approaches to pain management include pharmacological and non-pharmacological interventions. Non-pharmacological approaches to managing pain include physiotherapy for positioning and maintenance of function, heat pads or ice packs to reduce muscle aches, stiffness and oedema, and massage for relaxation (Lynch 2001). Relaxation and distraction therapies, hypnotherapy, transcutaneous electrical nerve stimulation (TENS) and acupuncture are other non-pharmacological approaches employed to manage pain (O'Hara 1996).

The use of drugs is an important component of pain management. Pharmacological interventions include systemic analgesic drugs, adjuvant drugs that 'help' more traditional analgesics, topical anaesthetics and analgesics, and drugs for specific conditions such as nitroglycerines for angina (Briggs 2002).

The World Health Organization analgesic ladder

The World Health Organization (WHO) analgesic ladder was introduced to improve pain control in patients with cancer pain (WHO 1986), although it also provides a framework for other types of pain management too. The WHO ladder embraces the combination of opioid, non-opioid and adjuvant medications. Adjuvants are drugs that are not usually analgesic themselves, but in combination with analgesic drugs may enhance the analgesic effect. There are three steps in the 'ladder', and they are only ascended when pain persists. The first step is to use non-opioid drugs like paracetamol or non-steroidal anti-inflammatory drugs (NSAIDs) with or without adjuvants, for mild pain. If the pain persists the second step is to introduce weak opioids like codeine with or without adjuvants. The final step of the ladder is ascended when pain continues and strong opioids such as morphine are introduced with or without non-opioid and adjuvant analgesia.

Non-opioid analgesia includes paracetamol and NSAIDs such as aspirin and ibuprofen. They exert their analgesic effect in the periphery by inhibiting prostaglandin synthesis and therefore the activation and sensitization of nociceptors (Barasi 1991). There is a limit or 'ceiling' to their analgesic efficacy beyond which increasing the dose will have no effect. The enzyme responsible for prostaglandin synthesis is cyclo-oxygenase (COX). Cyclo-oxygenase exists in two forms, COX-1 and COX-2. The COX-1 enzyme is important in homeostatic functions and COX-2 induces prostaglandins, which are involved in inflammation (Buttar & Wang 2000, Jordan & White 2001). Some NSAIDs selectively inhibit COX-2 without affecting COX-1 and may have fewer side effects (Buttar & Wang 2000).

Opioids are widely used in the management of somatic and visceral pain (Lynch 2001) and cancer pain (Harrison 2001). Weak opioids such as dihydrocodeine and codeine are used in step two of the WHO ladder, and strong opioids such as morphine and pethidine are used in step three. Opioids bind to specific receptors within the central nervous system. Opioid drugs (exogenous opioids) mimic the effects of naturally occurring opioids, the endorphins. Opioids produce analgesia by binding to opioid receptors and thereby modulating pain via the gating mechanism in the spinal cord. Opioid receptors are also found in certain sites in the brain including the periaqueductal grey matter (Barasi 1991). There is evidence that opioids also have peripheral effects since opioid receptors are located on peripheral terminals of sensory neurons (Stein et al 1995).

Opioids are available in a variety of formulations and can be administered via different routes. Doses are given incrementally until pain is effectively controlled or unwanted side effects occur: this is called titration, and is the adjustment of medication to achieve optimal analgesia. When these drugs are given at regular intervals, large fluctuations in blood levels are avoided, breakthrough pain is minimized and side effects are less likely. The key side effects of opioid drugs are nausea and vomiting, constipation and depression of breathing. Respiratory depression is rare if there has been effective titration of the dose (O'Hara 1996).

Patient-controlled analgesia (PCA), in which drugs are administered via an electronically controlled pump, is accepted as an important method of providing pain relief. A systematic review of randomized controlled trials of PCA using opioids to manage postoperative pain illustrated that patients prefer PCA over conventional analgesia and that the pain relief is more effective (Ballantyne et al 1993).

Adjuvant medications potentiate the analgesic effects of the opioids, which means that the opioid doses can be smaller and the incidence of side effects reduced.

Adjuvant drugs include antidepressants, anticonvulsants, muscle relaxants and corticosteroids (Hawthorn & Redmond 1998). The mechanism of action of antidepressants in pain relief is different from their role in lifting mood in depression (Wall 1999). Antidepressants lift mood by increasing serotonin levels (see Ch. 5). This same neurotransmitter is used in the descending inhibitory pathways and therefore antidepressants can offer pain relief. A systematic review of randomised controlled trials reveals that antidepressants were effective in reducing neuropathic pain (McQuay & Moore 1998).

In summary, pain is a complex multidimensional experience. Pain stimuli trigger nociceptors to fire off nerve impulses along nerve fibres to the spinal cord. A-delta fibres and C fibres carry pain information to the dorsal horn in the spinal cord. Here the relative activity of large diameter afferents carrying sensory information such as touch or warmth modulates the pain signals passing to the brain. The 'gate' tends to close when the activity in the large diameter afferents is greater than the activity in the pain fibres. When the activity in the small diameter pain fibres is greater, the 'gate' opens and more pain is felt. Descending pathways from the brain also exert effects on the gating mechanism in the spinal cord, which explains how psychological factors can influence the pain experience.

Introducing the spinal cord

The spinal cord is a very delicate structure that develops from the neural tube during fetal development. The spinal cord is part of the CNS linking the brain to the rest of the body. It stretches from the medulla oblongata in the brain through the centre of the vertebral column until it reaches the level of the second lumbar vertebra. There are 31 pairs of spinal nerves associated with the spinal cord, and together they carry incoming and outgoing signals to and from the brain.

The spinal cord lies within the vertebral canal, a space in the middle of the bony vertebral column. It is protected by the meninges and the small vertebrae, which encase it. The spinal cord is divided into regions or segments that relate to the vertebrae through which it passes. These are called the cervical, thoracic, lumbar and sacral segments.

There are two obvious enlargements found in the spinal cord: the cervical enlargement in the neck region, which gives rise to nerves in the arms, and the lumbar enlargement, which gives off nerves to the legs. The spinal cord narrows to a cone-like region called the conus medullaris, from where a collection of nerves arise, called the cauda equina or 'horses tails' (see Fig. 8.6).

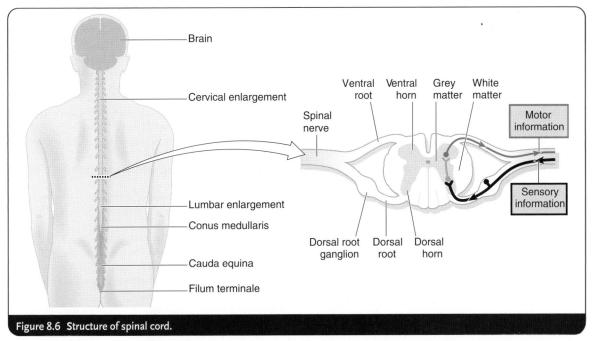

Figure 8.6 Structure of spinal cord.

Posterior view of spinal cord showing emergence of spinal nerves. The enlarged section of the spinal cord shows the arrangement of white and grey matter and the dorsal and ventral roots of the spinal nerves.

A cross-section of the spinal cord shows a core of grey matter in a butterfly shape surrounded by white matter. The 'wings' of the butterfly are called the dorsal and ventral horns. Spinal nerves contain both sensory and motor neurons; the sensory neurons carrying sensory information enter the spinal cord via the dorsal root, whilst the motor neurons leave the spinal cord via the ventral root carrying motor information to muscles and glands (see Fig. 8.6).

The spinal cord acts as an information highway between the brain and parts of the body, with information flowing in both directions. The white matter of the spinal cord is highly organized into columns of ascending and descending tracts. Ascending tracts carry sensory information from all over the body to the brain and descending tracts carry motor information from the brain to muscles and glands. Most tracts cross over, or decussate, at some point and they are always paired, with one tract on the left and another on the right side of the spinal cord. In addition, the grey matter is organized into a number of layers or lamina dealing with different types of information.

Another important function of the spinal cord is that it is the integrating centre for spinal reflexes. Spinal reflexes are automatic, unconscious responses to changes in the external or internal environment that are coordinated within the spinal cord. The responses result from nerve impulses being carried along relatively simple nerve pathways consisting of two or three neurons called a reflex arc. These responses help to maintain homeostasis.

References

Al-Chaer E D, Traub R J 2002 Biological basis of visceral pain: recent developments. Pain 96(3):221–225

Astley A 1990 A history of pain. Nursing 4(17):33–35

Ballantyne J C, Carr D B, Chalmers T C et al 1993 Postoperative patient-controlled analgesia: meta-analyses of initial randomised control trials. Journal of Clinical Anesthesia 5:182–193

Barasi S 1991 The physiology of pain. Surgical Nurse 4(5):14–20

Bernard J F, Besson J M 1990 The spino (Trigemino) pontoamygdaloid pathway: electrophysiological evidence for involvement in pain processes. Journal of Neurophysiology 63:473–490

Breen J 2002 Transitions in the concept of pain. Advances in Nursing Science 24(4):48–59

Briggs E 2002 The nursing management of pain in older people. Nursing Older People 14(7):23–29

Buttar N S, Wang K K 2002 The 'Aspirin' of the new millennium: cyclooxygenase-2 inhibitors. Mayo Clinical Proceedings 75(10):1027–1038

Carr D B, Goudas L C 1999 Acute pain. Lancet 353(9169):2051–2058

Casey K L 1996 Match and mismatch: identifying the neuronal determinants of pain. Annals of Internal Medicine 124(11):995–998

Cross S A 1994 Pathophysiology of pain. Mayo Clinical Proceedings 69:375–383

Derbyshire S W G 2002 Measuring our natural painkiller. Trends in Neuroscience 25(2):67–68

Dickenson A H 1995 Central acute pain mechanisms. Annals of Medicine 27(2):223–227

Haigh R C, Blake D R 2001 Understanding pain. Clinical Medicine 1(1):44–48

Harrison P 2001 Update on pain management for advanced genitourinary cancer. Journal of Urology 165(1):1849–1858

Hawthorn J, Redmond K 1998 Pain: Causes and management. Blackwell Science, Oxford

IASP subcommittee on taxonomy 1979 Pain terms: a list with definitions and notes on usage. Pain 6:247–252

Jackson A 1995 Acute pain: its physiology and the pharmacology of analgesia. Nursing Times 91(16):27–28

Jordan S, White J 2001 Non-steroidal anti-inflammatory drugs: clinical issues. Nursing Standard 15(23):45–52

Liu H, Mantyh P W, Basbaum A I 1997 NMDA-receptor regulation of substance P release from primary afferent nociceptors. Nature 386(6626):721–724

Lynch M 2001 Pain as the fifth vital sign. Journal of Intravenous Nursing 24(2):85–94

McCaffery M, Pasero C 1999 Pain: Clinical manual. Mosby, St Louis

McHugh J M, McHugh W B 2000 Pain: neuroanatomy, chemical mediators, and clinical implications. AACN Clinical Issues 11(2):168–178

McQuay H J, Moore R A 1998 An evidenced-based resource for pain relief. Oxford University Press, Oxford

Melzack R 1973 The puzzle of pain. Penguin, Harmondsworth, p 49

Melzak R, Wall P D 1965 Pain mechanisms: a new theory. Science 150:971–979

Merskey H 1986 Classification of chronic pain. Descriptions of chronic pain syndromes and definitions of pain terms. Pain (Supplement 3):51–225

Merskey H 1994 Pain and psychological medicine. In: Wall P, Melzack R (eds) Textbook of pain, 3rd edn. Churchill Livingstone, Edinburgh, p 903–920

Monafo W W 1995 Physiology of pain. Journal of Burn Care & Rehabilitation 16(3):345–347

Motluk A 1999 Ouch! That hurt. New Scientist 162(2185):17

O'Hara P 1996 Pain management for health professionals. Chapman and Hall, London

Price D D 1995 Unpleasant pain evoked by thalamic stimulation. Nature Medicine 1(9):885–887

Rey R 1995 The history of pain. Harvard University Press, London

Ren K, Dubner R 2002 Descending modulation in persistent pain: an update. Pain 100:1–6

Roberge C, McEwen M 1998 The effects of local anaesthetics on postoperative pain. AORN Journal 68(6):1003–1012

Stein C, Schafer M, Hassan A H 1995 Peripheral opioid receptors. Annals of Medicine 27(2):219–221

Treede R D 1995 Peripheral acute pain mechanisms. Annals of Medicine 27(2):213–216

Wall P 1999 Pain: the science of suffering. Weidenfield & Nicholson, London

Wilson M 2002 Overcoming the challenges of neuropathic pain. Nursing Standard 16(33):47–53

Woolf C J 1995 How to hit pain before it hurts you. MRC News 67:17–21

Woolf C J, Salter M W 2000 Neuronal plasticity: Increasing the gain in pain. Science 288(5472):1765–1768

World Health Organization 1986 Cancer pain relief. WHO, Geneva

Youngson R 1992 Pathways to pain control. New Scientist 133(1813):30–33

9
GROWTH

A woman's skin was a map of the town where she'd grown from a child. When she went out, she covered it up with a dress, with a shawl, with a hat, with mitts or a muff, with leggings, trousers or jeans, with an ankle-length cloak, hooded and fingertip-sleeved. But – birthmark, tattoo – the A–Z street map grew, a precise second skin, broad if she binged, thin when she slimmed, a précis of where to end or go back or begin.

(Carol Ann Duffy 2002)

The adult human body contains about 50 million, million cells, all developed from a single cell, the fertilized ovum. This tremendous increase in numbers results from individual cells dividing over and over again. The mechanism of enlargement from a single cell to a multi-cellular organism is a complicated business. Before cells divide, chromosomes reproduce themselves so that each daughter cell contains exactly the same genetic information as the parent cell. Humans, like all other living organisms, grow from metabolic processes, the food we eat contains all kinds of chemical substances that are taken in, broken down and reassembled into new building materials.

Growth describes an increase in size such as the increase in height or weight of a child. However, a baby does not resemble the fertilized egg from which it arose. All the changes that lead from an undifferentiated state to a highly organized, specialized and mature state are described as development (Bogin 1999). Changes through the human life cycle reflect both growth and development and comprise three features: an increase in size, differentiation of structure and function, and a change in form.

The principles of human growth and development can be introduced by examining some of the processes, phases and patterns that contribute to the human life cycle. The growth and development of an embryo illustrates some of these principles.

From simple beginnings

The fertilized ovum is called a zygote and undergoes substantial growth and development before it becomes an embryo. During embryonic growth and development the zygote, a single cell, divides into tens of thousands of new cells. In the first few cell divisions, exact copies of the parent cell form; by the end of the second week different groups of cells begin to develop, ultimately resulting in the cell specializations necessary for the formation of a mature adult.

Following fertilization, the zygote divides several times as it travels down the fallopian tube towards the uterus, which has been prepared to become a favourable environment for growth and development. During these very early stages of human growth and development the cellular processes of growth, multiplication, movement and differentiation are at their simplest and most easy to understand.

Cells reproduce by dividing into two; so the fertilized ovum divides into two, these two cells divide into four and so on until a solid ball of cells called the morula forms. Cell movement then begins and the cells arrange themselves into an irregular hollow ball called the blastocyst, consisting of about a hundred cells (Leese 1989). The blastocyst implants into the thickened lining of the uterus, the endometrium, by the end of the first week (Bee 1994). More elaborate organization then occurs with the formation of the inner cell mass, which eventually forms the fetus. The other cells develop into tissues that support the embryo, such as the placenta (Monk 1992). The embryonic disc develops from the inner cell mass and by the beginning of the third week, in a process called gastrulation, has transformed into three germ layers (see Fig. 9.1). These eventually lead to the specialization of cells and tissues necessary for the new individual to grow and develop through the various stages of the human life cycle.

Of the three distinct germ layers, the ectoderm develops into the skin, mucous membranes and the nervous system; the mesoderm forms the basis for the musculoskeletal system and several internal organs; and the endoderm gives rise to the digestive system (Monk 1992). The development of organs and physiological

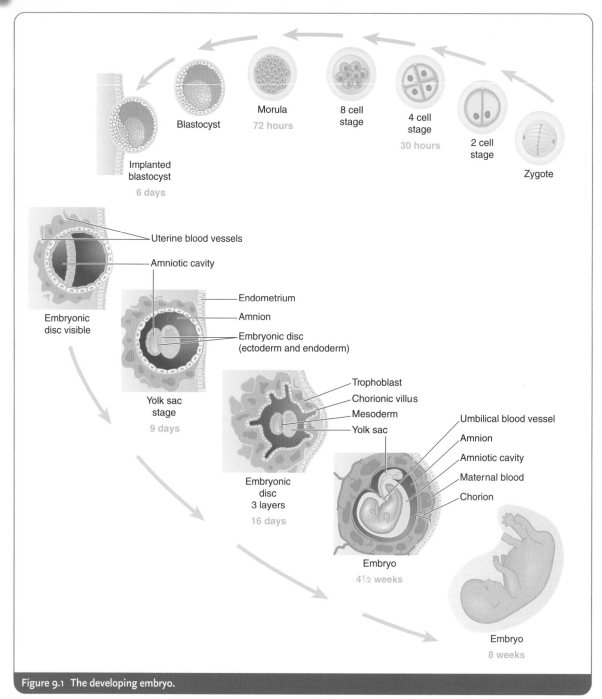

Figure 9.1 The developing embryo.

Events prior to implantation and after the blastocyst has implanted are shown. The three layers of the embryonic disc give rise to specialization of cells and tissues in the human form, which is clearly recognizable at eight weeks.

systems of the embryo during the next few weeks is called organogenesis (Bogin 1999).

The nervous system begins to develop during the third week from a section of the ectoderm, the neural plate. Movement of cells in the neural plate leads to the development of a neural groove and then a neural crest. The neural crest bulges, enlarges and eventually forms the neural tube, which becomes the brain and spinal cord.

During embryonic development there are certain critical periods in the formation of organs which are particularly sensitive to any disturbance. Any agent that causes disruption to the development of the embryo or fetus is called a teratogen (Polifka & Friedman 2002). Teratogenic exposures can disrupt prenatal development in a number of ways, including changes in programmed cell death (apoptosis), cell migration, proliferation and alterations in gene expression (Polifka & Friedman 2002). The gestational timing of the exposure and nature of the agent are instrumental in determining its impact (Rubin 1998).

Neural tube defects

Defects may arise if the neural tube fails to close during the third and fourth week of gestation. Both environmental factors and a genetic predisposition are implicated in babies born with spina bifida or anencephaly. Low levels of folic acid are associated with these neural tube defects and folic acid supplementation prior to conception has reduced their incidence (Hasenau & Covington 2002, Polifka & Friedman 2002). Women are encouraged to take folic acid prior to conception and during the first 12 weeks of gestation (Seaman 1997, Barrowclough & Ford 2000). Increased levels of homocysteine are a risk factor for neural tube defects and folic acid is protective because it contributes to the metabolism of homocysteine (Hasenau & Covington 2002).

Cell movement and programmed cell death

Growth and development of the embryo is achieved by the processes of cell division, allocation of cells to different lineages, cell differentiation, cell movement (Monk 1992, Cooke 1995) and programmed cell death (Raff 1995). The importance of cell movement in the developing embryo is illustrated by the neural crest cells. These cells migrate in defined routes, giving rise not only to the nervous system as outlined above, but also skin pigmentation and cartilages in the jaw and neck (Cooke 1995). Complex cell movements and interactions between shifting populations of cells are necessary in the developing embryo.

Programmed cell death or apoptosis is also crucial in development; many structures form that are later removed by apoptosis (Meier et al 2000). Apoptosis is seen in the development of the hand, which begins as a paddle-like structure with the fingers becoming defined as the cells between them die (Raff 1995,

Wallis 1997). Apoptosis is also a mechanism for getting rid of damaged cells, and suppression of apoptosis contributes to the development of cancer cells (Evan & Vousden 2001). The architecture of tissues in the body is due to the processes of cell proliferation, differentiation and demolition or programmed cell death (Meier et al 2000).

Cell differentiation

Cells do not just divide during embryonic development, they also become differentiated or specialized. During the first few cell divisions all of the cells are the same and they retain the capability of developing into a whole organism. These cells are called multi-potent cells. As the embryo develops, the cells quickly become committed to certain cell lineages. Eventually, about a hundred different kinds of specialized cells form, each having a different role in homeostasis. Each cell, with some exceptions, contains the same complement of genes as those in the original zygote from which they developed (Monk 1992). This means that, during development, different genes in differentiated cells are switched on or off. This is termed gene expression (see p. 130). The mechanisms that regulate gene expression during growth and development of the embryo are not fully known, but include hormones and various growth factors (Evans 1994, Sinclair & Dangerfield 1998).

Stem cells have the capability to transform and replenish the different tissue types that make up the body and they also represent the fundamental building blocks of human development. There are two broad categories of stem cells: adult (somatic) stem cells and embryonic stem cells. Embryonic stem cells are considered to have huge potential in basic research and, eventually, clinical applications, although there are many ethical and legal issues to be considered (Pedersen 1999, Gepstein 2002). In adults, haemopoietic stem cells in bone marrow transplants have the capacity to form the basis for the complete haemopoietic system (Stanworth & Newland 2001).

Cell growth, division and the cell cycle

Cell division, or mitosis, contributes to homeostasis in a number of ways. The continuing process of cell division ensures that a single cell grows into a human adult steadily and gradually, enabling homeostasis to be maintained in all stages. In mitosis, crucial genetic material containing the blueprint for life and homeostasis is transmitted from one cell to another. Mitosis is also responsible for the replacement of worn out or damaged cells to ensure optimum tissue functioning. Cell differentiation leads to development of different cell lineages and, ultimately, the tissues and organs that function together to maintain homeostasis.

Some cells in the body continue to undergo cell division in adulthood. These include blood cells and epithelial cells such as those that line the gut; these are renewing tissues. Other cells such as nerve cells and skeletal muscle are incapable of dividing once they have differentiated during development; these are called static tissues. There are still other, expanding, tissues, in which cells do not divide unless cells are destroyed; cells in the liver and kidney, for example, remain capable of proliferating (Bogin 1999, Hyams 2002).

The cell cycle

The cell cycle is responsible for dictating the life of the cell and the timing of when and if it divides (Nurse

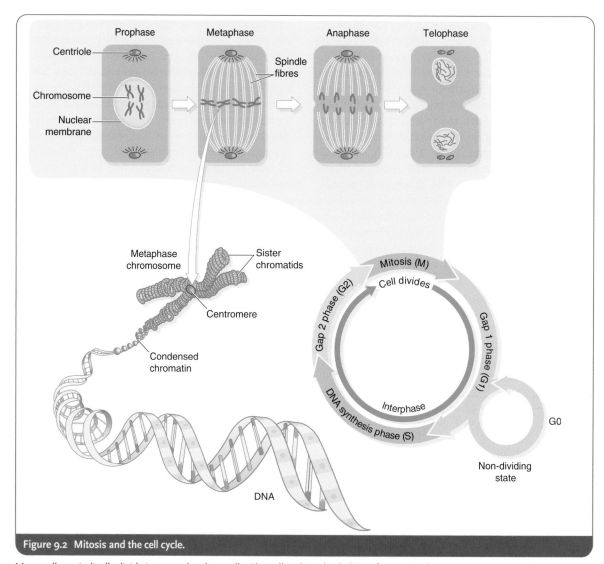

Figure 9.2 Mitosis and the cell cycle.

Many cells periodically divide into two daughter cells. The cell cycle is divided into four main phases. During mitosis the chromosomes separate so that each daughter cell receives identical copies of the replicated DNA. The drawings show two chromosome pairs for simplicity, in humans there are 23 pairs.

1999). Each time a cell divides, the DNA within it is duplicated and then the double set of chromosomes must be divided equally between the two daughter cells. Exact replication and division of DNA is essential to pass accurate genetic instructions to subsequent daughter cells. The cell cycle ensures this is carried out precisely and in the correct sequence (Hyams 2002).

The cell cycle is a series of events (see Fig. 9.2) that occurs between cell formation and division into two daughter cells. Interphase is the part of the cell cycle that lies between divisions and different cells can remain in interphase for variable lengths of time – hours, weeks or years (Gull 1996). Interphase is made up of the G1, S and G2 phases of the cell cycle (Hyams 2002). In the first gap phase, G1, the cell makes the decision to replicate DNA. In the second gap, G2, the cell grows and ensures that DNA replication is complete before mitosis begins (Gull 1996). When a cell is in a non-dividing state it resides in the G0 state. During the S phase DNA is replicated (see p. 128). The two identical copies of DNA, the sister chromatids, are joined together by a centromere forming the familiar X-shaped chromosomes seen during mitosis. Cell division involves two processes: mitosis, which ensures that equal and exact copies of the chromosomes are distributed to the daughter cells, and cytokinesis, which is the division or cleavage of cytoplasm into two cells.

Mitosis

There are four phases in mitosis which describe the pattern of chromosome movements (see Fig. 9.2) (Bickmore 1995). During the first stage (called the prophase), the DNA, with associated proteins called chromatin, becomes tightly coiled, or condensed. The two newly formed pairs of centrioles move to opposite sides of the cytoplasm, and the nuclear membrane and nucleoli break down and disappear. Microtubules become associated with the centrioles and the spindle apparatus begins to form (Gull 1996).

Metaphase is a key stage in mitosis. In this, the chromosomes, consisting of two sister chromatids, jostle for space around the middle of the spindle apparatus. Each chromatid becomes attached to a spindle fibre, which runs from the centromere to one of the poles of the spindle. Each of the 46 chromosomes with its two identical chromatids is at the centre of a carefully balanced tug of war, in which each chromatid is delicately poised before being pulled to opposite poles of the spindle (Bickmore 1998).

During anaphase, the spindle fibres shorten, causing the chromatids to start to be pulled apart (Gull 1996). In telophase, the separated chromosomes group together at opposite poles of the spindle, and the chromosomes begin to unwind and become threadlike structures. Next, a nuclear membrane forms around each set of chromosomes, nucleoli appear within the new nuclei and the microtubules disappear (Gull 1996). Finally, the cytoplasm divides by cytokinesis and two separate cells are formed (Bickmore 1998).

Signals for cell division

Long-lived organisms such as humans have to be able to engage in cell proliferation throughout life to support development, cell renewal and repair. Cell division must be accurate, controlled and coordinated during the journey through the life cycle (see Fig. 9.3); this is achieved by a series of control pathways that respond to signals inside and outside the cell (Carr 1995). Control over cell proliferation is crucial to make sure that homeostasis is maintained and cancer is avoided (Carr 1995, Hyams 2002).

At a point in G1, called 'Start', the decision is made whether to complete the cell cycle. If the external signals are unfavourable the cell can exit into the quiescent non-dividing state called G0 or leave the cycle at Start to differentiate into a specialized cell (Hyams 2002). When the signals are right the cell crosses the G1/S border and is committed to completing the cell cycle.

A group of enzymes called the cyclin-dependent protein kinases (CDKs) are vital to the control of the cell cycle (Nurse 1999). These enzymes are dependent on a protein called cyclin to function correctly. This protein fluctuates throughout the cell cycle and activates the cyclin-dependent protein kinases when it reaches a critical level. One of these enzymes, called CDK1, coupled with a particular cyclin is considered to be the master switch that controls cell cycle events (Hyams 2002).

During the cell cycle there are two checkpoints. The first ensures that the DNA is not damaged, and the second checks that the mitotic spindle formation and attachment of chromosomes to it are correct. These checks ensure that mutations are relatively rare and block the progression of any damaged cells through the cell cycle (Hyams 2002). Failure of these cell cycle control mechanisms leads to the inappropriate cell divisions that cause cancer (see Ch. 10) (Carr 1995). Cancer cells ignore the stop and start signals and their

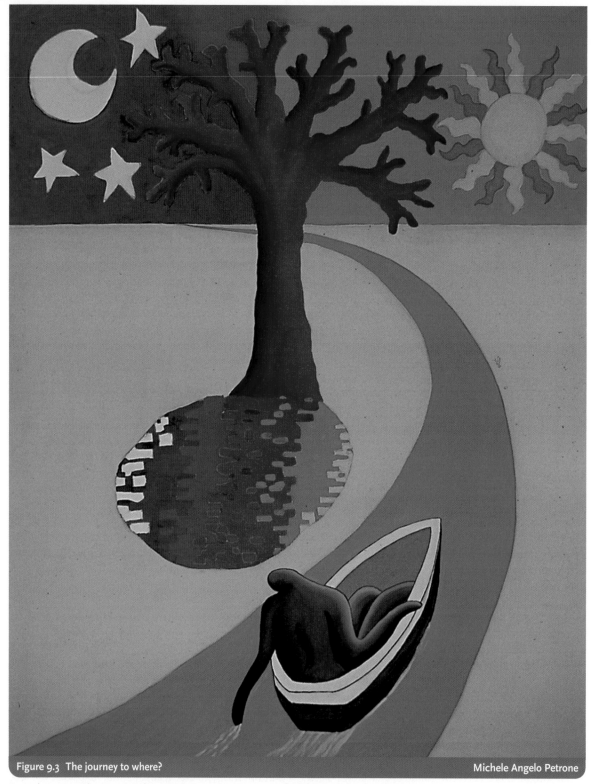

Figure 9.3 The journey to where?

Michele Angelo Petrone

From the series 'The Emotional Cancer Journey' (see www.mapfoundation.org). This is a series of paintings depicting the artist's own illness, Hodgkin's disease (cancer of the lymph glands), diagnosed in 1994. (Reproduced with kind permission of the artist.)

proliferation becomes uncontrolled and tumours can develop (Hyams 2002).

Patterns of growth

There are four main phases in human growth. In the early embryo the key focus is cell multiplication rather than cell differentiation. As the embryo develops, there is a balance between growth and differentiation; this phase continues throughout childhood and ends at maturity. During adulthood cell growth is directed towards cell renewal. Finally, in the last phase, during senescence, cell renewal does not match cell loss. This causes tissues to be less efficient and homeostasis is more difficult to maintain (Sinclair & Dangerfield 1998).

At birth a baby measures about 50 cm in length, which is about 5000 times longer than the ovum. The baby then grows about three and half times in length to reach adult height; this illustrates that growth is not uniform throughout the life cycle (Sinclair and Dangerfield 1998). Studies of internal organs demonstrate that there are different patterns to their growth (Bogin 1999). For example, the nervous system grows rapidly in childhood; by about 6 years, the nervous system is about 90% of adult size. The growth of reproductive organs is very slow until puberty when their growth increases dramatically (Sinclair and Dangerfield 1998, Bogin 1999).

Determinants of growth

The growth of a child is determined by a complex interaction of genes, hormones and environmental factors. Genes inherited from parents are important since tall families usually have tall children and smaller children tend to have smaller parents. This is because we inherit many different genes that affect the size and shape of the body, including those that control the development of the long bones. Nutrition and other environmental factors also have a significant influence on growth and development. The secular trends in height are linked to improvements in standards of living and nutrition and this illustrates the influence of socio-economic factors on adult height (Spencer & Logan 2002). Other factors that influence growth during childhood include altitude, climate, seasons and month of birth (Sinclair & Dangerfield 1998, Bogin 1999).

Nutrition

An adequate supply of nutrients is needed to grow and develop normally. The calorie intake required for optimal growth and development varies during the human life cycle. Children need a high energy diet to support the rapid growth of their brains. Somewhere between 40–85% of the resting metabolism is used to maintain the brain compared to 16–25% in adults (Leonard & Robertson 1994). Apart from calories, the range and amount of various nutrients is important and this includes macronutrients such as protein, carbohydrate and fat, but also a range of micronutrients including vitamins, minerals and trace elements.

There are two long chain polyunsaturated fatty acids (PUFAs) that are thought to be very important for both fetal and infant development; these are omega-6 (arachidonic acid) and omega-3 (docosahexaenoic acid) fatty acids (Turner 2001). Omega-3 and omega-6 are significant components of the brain, nervous system, retina, blood vessels and many other cells and organs. These two PUFAs make up more than 30% of brain lipids and brain lipids contribute to 60% of brain tissue (Turner 2001). These essential fatty acids are found naturally in breast milk and are one of the many reasons breast feeding may be advantageous for cognitive and visual function (Gordon 1997). Most formula feeds contain low levels or lack PUFAs altogether; when these fatty acids are added to formula milk they seem to improve mental development (Josefson 2000).

Nutrition during fetal growth and development may also influence the health of the individual in adult life. Some studies have suggested links between poor fetal growth and later cardiovascular disease. Sub-optimum nutrition in pregnancy, leading to malnutrition in the fetus during a critical period, may be instrumental in increasing the likelihood of hypertension, coronary heart disease and type 2 diabetes in adult life (Gordon 1997, Phillips 2002). The hypothesis that adult disease has fetal origins suggests that malnutrition at a critical time could permanently alter or programme growth and development of the cardiovascular system (Barker 2001). The role of fetal hormones, particularly those of the HPA axis (see p. 70), are being investigated as likely mediators of the programming of cardiovascular disease in adult life (Green 2001, Phillips 2002). Nutritional programming in babies is also being investigated for its influence on long-term health and learning abilities (Lucas 1996).

Genes

Genetic control of growth is polygenic, which means many genes are involved (see p. 134). These genes each produce small additive influences that shape the potential for growth. Genes, the proteins they produce, and hormones interact in determining growth and development. One particular group of genes, called homeobox genes, are thought to play a key role in development and differentiation (Castronovo et al 1994). The homeobox genes code for proteins that control the pattern of expression of other genes (Wallis 1997). Genes are especially important in shaping the different male and female patterns of growth. Up to the age of about ten years, the growth patterns of girls and boys are similar although not identical. The difference in timing and intensity of the adolescent growth spurt is responsible for the different size of adult men and women (Sinclair & Dangerfield 1998). This onset of the adolescent growth spurt is mainly controlled by genetic factors, although hormonal and environment factors also play a role. The adolescent growth spurt seems to be a unique feature of human growth and development (Bogin 1999).

Hormones

Most hormones influence growth, but there are several major hormones that are particularly influential, including thyroid hormones, gonadal hormones, adrenal hormones and growth hormone (Sinclair & Dangerfield 1998). Thyroid hormones are important for the growth and development of bones, teeth and the brain (see p. 47). Cortisol, the stress hormone (see p. 70), actually opposes growth by stimulating protein breakdown and inhibiting bone growth. It also has a marked influence on the distribution of body fat. Increased cortisol secretion may contribute to the impaired growth of children with chronic illness. Long-term steroid therapy can also have an adverse impact on a child's growth (Sharek & Bergman 2000, Simon et al 2001).

Growth hormone

Growth hormone (GH) is secreted from the anterior pituitary gland and is one of the most important hormones for determining growth in childhood. Human growth hormone (hGH) is not essential for fetal growth. The key factor in fetal and infant growth is nutrition and it is only during the latter part of infancy that hGH becomes the main controller of the rate of human growth and development (Sinclair & Dangerfield 1998).

Human growth hormone has a key role in stimulating DNA synthesis, cell division and growth in height during childhood. Growth in long bones relies on the presence of epiphyseal plates or discs found towards the ends of long bones. These growth plates contain cartilage cells that are actively dividing; proliferation of these cartilage cells is stimulated by hGH. Once the epiphyseal plates disappear, long bones cannot grow in length and hGH no longer has an effect on longitudinal growth.

GH secretion is stimulated by GH-releasing hormone and inhibited by somatostatin operating via negative feedback loops (Shalet 2000). GH secretion follows a circadian rhythm (see Ch. 7) with highest levels being secreted during sleep (Van Cauter & Plat 1996). Apart from during sleep, GH secretion is enhanced following exercise and when blood glucose levels are low (Shalet 2000). The pulses of GH secretion during sleep help to explain why sleep is good for healing (see Ch. 7) (Hodgson 1991). Whilst GH secretion is at its highest during puberty, it is the sex steroid hormones, oestrogen and testosterone, that are responsible for the adolescent growth spurt (Shalet 2000). GH secretion starts to wane after puberty, although GH continues to exert important effects on metabolism in adult life.

GH therapy can be given to children with a GH insufficiency to enhance their growth and adult height. The use of GH therapy in children of short stature, but who do not have GH deficiency, is controversial. Under these circumstances, the GH supplements may be offered to short normal children in the belief that they are socially or psychologically disadvantaged (Voss 1999, Shalet 2000). GH deficiency in adults is associated with a number of characteristics, including weight gain, changes in body composition, decreased bone mass and an increased risk of cardiovascular disease (Shalet 2000). Evidence for the efficacy of GH replacement therapy in adults with GH deficiency is inconclusive and the long-term benefits and risks are not yet known (Isley 2002).

Many of the effects of growth hormone are mediated through somatomedins or insulin-like growth factors (IGFs) which are produced in a number of tissues, especially the liver (Shalet 2000). The IGFs are similar in structure to insulin, hence their name. IGF-1 is an important growth hormone that not only mediates the effects of GH, but also exerts an independent growth-promoting effect (Laron 2001).

Growing older

During the latter part of the human life cycle the pattern of growth changes such that during old age, or senescence, cell renewal does not match cell loss. This has a number of consequences on capacity of tissues to maintain homeostasis. The pattern of ageing varies dramatically between individuals resulting from the interaction of many genes and environmental factors; ageing is a multifactorial phenomenon. Specific ageing changes occur in molecules, cells and organs, but they do not occur in all individuals and there is no predictable pattern to the ageing process (Bogin 1999).

There are many mechanisms that contribute to ageing, including DNA mutations, changes in mitochondrial function, damage by oxygen free radicals and accumulation of ageing proteins. Most theories of ageing incorporate the concept that ageing results from the accumulation of unrepaired damage. The cumulative and interactive nature of these ageing changes lead to functional deterioration, reduced capacity to cope with stress, and an increased incidence of chronic disease (Khaw 1997).

Disposable soma theory

This theory provides a framework for current ideas about the biology of ageing. It proposes that, in evolutionary terms, there is a tension between investing in the short-term maintenance of the soma (body tissues) against investing in reproduction and the viability of the germ line (eggs and sperm) over many generations. This theory proposes that organisms exposed to high risk have shorter lives and invest little in maintenance and a lot in reproduction. Conversely, organisms exposed to low risk that live longer have evolved more sophisticated maintenance systems. Cells from long-lived species are better protected against challenge from chemicals and other stresses than cells from animals that have shorter lifespans (Kirkwood 1999, Kirkwood 2002). Cells of the body are considered 'disposable', as long as the DNA in germ cells is intact and is passed on.

Whilst humans have good repair systems, they cannot cope with the cumulative damage that occurs over a lifetime. Human genes collectively do not invest enough in the maintenance of cells and tissues. Many genes contribute to ageing, although their number and relative importance have yet to be elucidated (Lithgow 1998).

Theories that suggest ageing results from the accumulation of random damage at the cell and molecular level are compatible with the disposable soma theory. Free radicals play a key role in the biological ageing process and oxidative stress is responsible for damage to cells (Lithgow 1998, Miquel 2001). Free radicals or reactive oxygen species (ROS) are also important contributors to dementia, heart disease and age-related blindness, which are more common in later life (Kirkwood 2002).

Free radicals are chemical by-products generated during the breaking down of oxygen. They accumulate with time and can damage DNA, proteins and cell membranes. Increased free radical production and damage is associated with a short lifespan, whereas humans have relatively low levels of oxidative stress and therefore have a longer lifespan. The influence of free radicals on longevity can be illustrated by comparing rats with pigeons, which live for about 35 years, or approximately 12 times as long as rats! Pigeons and rats are about the same size and consume similar amounts of oxygen, but pigeons produce less free radicals than rats do (Hopkin 1999). A diet containing adequate amounts of antioxidants, which disable free radicals, can help to protect against tissue damage caused by ROS. Antioxidants are found in fruits, vegetables, green tea; they are in fact vitamins A, C and E, selenium (a mineral), and a group known as the carotenoids. Eating enough antioxidants in the diet helps to preserve health in old age (Miquel 2001).

Telomeres and ageing

The ends of chromosomes are protected by telomeres (Kirkwood 1999). The inability of somatic cells to carry on dividing forever is due to the shortening of telomeres (Kirkwood 2002). Each time a cell divides the telomeres shorten by about 100 base pairs and this enables telomeres to monitor how many times the cell divides (Kipling & Faragher 1999). When the telomeres become too short, the cells stop dividing, but how telomere shortening brings about cell senescence remains a mystery (Brown 1998). Cell senescence is a state in which cells are living, but no longer capable of dividing (Kipling & Faragher 1999). Oxidative damage is an important factor in shortening telomeres, reinforcing the significance of free radicals and telomere shortening in the ageing process (Kirkwood 2002).

The role of telomere shortening and cell ageing may be an important factor in the premature ageing of Dolly the cloned sheep. Cloning animals is accomplished by transferring a somatic cell nucleus into an ovum that has had its own nucleus removed. Genes in the donor nucleus are reprogrammed by the cytoplasm in the ovum and the cell proceeds to develop into an embryo and ultimately mature adult (Kühholzer-Cabot & Brem 2002). Dolly aged prematurely and suffered from arthritis (Williams 2002). There is some indication that cloned sheep may have excessive telomere shortening reflecting the age of the donor sheep and this leads to ageing effects at a younger chronological age (Kühholzer-Cabot & Brem 2002).

Ageing, homeostasis and health

Ageing results from the accumulation of random molecular damage over many decades. Mutations in the mitochondrial DNA acquired during life are implicated in ageing and neurodegenerative diseases (see p. 8) (Walker 1994, Wallace 1999, Kirkwood 2000). The damage caused to cells and their lack of replacement results in some organs losing their functional reserve. Ageing is seen most obviously in non-dividing cells. Cells found in the core of the lens are as old as the individual and the ageing proteins within them can cause cataracts (Hipkiss 1994).

There is a distinction between diseases associated with old age and changes that are due to the ageing process (Green 1994). Diseases that contribute to secondary ageing include atherosclerosis, type 2 diabetes, essential hypertension and osteoporosis (Holloszy 2000). Often the diseases are mistaken for ageing changes or there is blurring between the two (Andrews 2001).

Individual changes that occur in different organ systems need to be considered together rather than separately since compensatory changes may occur (Herbert 1991). Each physiological system has a spare capacity. Only when the functional capacity can no longer meet homeostatic needs do problems occur.

Ageing is influenced by a variety of stressors, lifestyles and social support systems. There are many possible interventions for successful ageing. In terms of the biology of ageing, key strategies to consider are: diets low in fat and energy, high in fruit, vegetable content and antioxidants; exercise and hormone replacement (Holloszy 2000). A number of factors are also important for maintaining brain health, such as engaging in activities that are intellectually stimulating (Small 2002).

Introducing the reproductive systems

The combined functions of the reproductive systems are to produce sperm and ova; to transfer sperm to the female; to enable fertilization to occur; and to offer a suitable environment for the growth and development of the embryo and fetus. Human reproduction depends on the integrated action of hormones, and the nervous and reproductive systems.

The male reproductive system

The male reproductive system consists of the primary sex organs, the testes, several ducts, glands and the penis (see Fig. 9.4). Testes are suspended outside the abdominal cavity by the scrotum, a pouch of skin that has an arrangement of muscles that can hold the testes at varying distances from the body in order to maintain an optimal temperature for sperm development.

Each testis is divided into 200–300 wedge-shaped lobules; each of these contains coiled seminiferous tubules measuring about 250 metres in total. This is the site where sperm are produced at the rate of up to 300 million per day in a process called spermatogenesis. Spermatocytes develop from spermatogonia inside the seminiferous tubules and then divide by meiosis to produce spermatids that in turn develop into mature sperm (see Fig. 9.5). Sertoli cells are thought to support the development of the germ cells.

The secretion of testosterone from interstitial cells (Leydig cells) and maturation of sperm are controlled by hormones from the anterior pituitary gland. The anterior pituitary gland produces follicle-stimulating hormone (FSH) and luteinizing hormone (LH). Secretion of FSH and LH is controlled by the gonadotrophin-releasing hormone (GnRH) from the hypothalamus. Negative feedback by testosterone controls the actions of GnRH.

Glands and ducts

Sperm complete their development in another long coiled tube, the epididymis, before ejaculation. A series of ducts then convey sperm to the outside of the body. Various secretions are added on the way to provide the optimum environment for sperm (see Fig. 9.4). A duct called the vas deferens travels from each testis, and just before the prostate gland they fuse together to

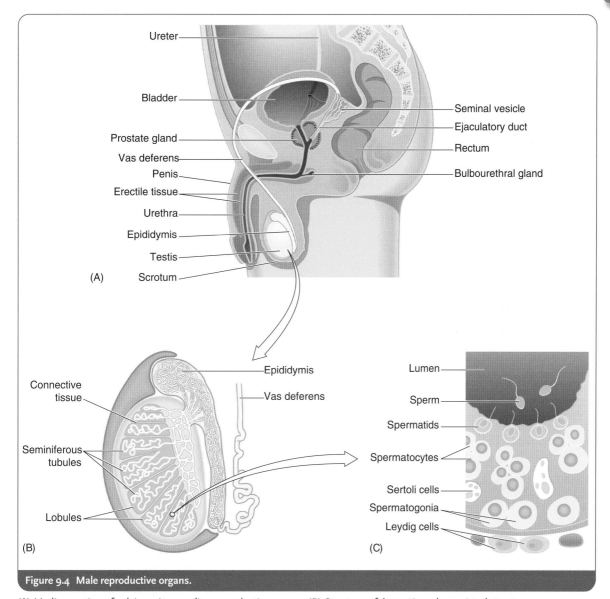

Figure 9.4 Male reproductive organs.

(A) Median section of pelvic cavity revealing reproductive organs. (B) Structure of the testis and associated structures. (C) Seminiferous tubule highly magnified illustrating development of sperm.

form the ejaculatory duct. This leads into the urethra, which passes through the penis. The urethra is responsible for carrying both urine and semen to the outside of the body. Alkaline secretions from the seminal vesicles, located just behind the prostate gland, add fructose and prostaglandins to sperm as they pass into the ejaculatory duct. The prostate gland secretes a milky fluid containing chemicals that stimulate sperm motility. The prostate gland varies in size during the human life cycle; it grows rapidly in size at puberty then remains fairly static during adulthood until middle age, when it often enlarges due to the effects of the changing balance of hormones and growth factors (Untergasser et al 1999). The bulbourethral gland secretes a mucus-like fluid that provides lubrication for intercourse. Sperm and the combined secretions, mainly seminal fluid, make up semen, which is slightly alkaline to offset the acidic environment of the vagina.

Spermatogenesis

Sperm production begins at puberty and continues throughout life. There are three phases in the production of sperm. The early phase involves cell division by mitosis to produce many spermatogonia and then further mitotic divisions to produce spermatocytes. The second phase is meiosis; the spermatocytes divide by meiosis to produce spermatids with only half the usual number of chromosomes. Each diploid 'parent' cell divides into four haploid daughter cells containing a single set of 23 chromosomes. The final phase called spermiogenesis then follows in which the round spermatids change into spermatozoa by developing a head and a tail (see Fig. 9.5) (Dudley 1995).

Spermatogenesis is controlled by LH and FSH. LH stimulates interstitial cells (Leydig cells) to secrete testosterone. Testosterone is considered important in maintaining spermatogenesis. FSH acts on Sertoli cells which, in response, synthesize proteins that are thought to signal germ cells to develop into sperm (Chantler 2003).

Meiosis

In spermatogenesis and oogenesis the nuclear material divides by meiosis. The key features of meiosis are that there are two cell divisions with no intervening DNA replication; this results in a halving of the chromosome number with daughter cells receiving a single set of 23 chromosomes. A key principle of meiosis is creating genetic diversity in the gametes. This is achieved via two mechanisms in the first meiotic division, called 'crossing-over' and random assortment. In the second meiotic division the chromosomes behave in a similar fashion as in mitosis (see p. 113).

Genetic diversity in germ cells

There are a number of stages in the division of chromosomes in meiosis. Prophase in the first meiotic division (prophase 1) is a long and complicated stage and is divided into a number of subdivisions (Baker 1992). DNA replication occurs prior to the first meiotic division during interphase. Each chromosome then consists of two identical chromatids.

Homologous chromosomes (see p. 128) come together in pairs in prophase 1, forming a four-stranded

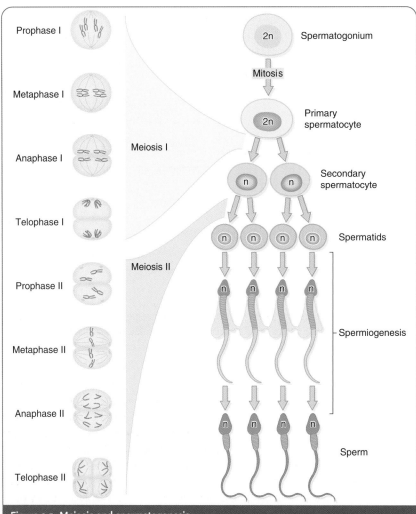

Figure 9.5 Meiosis and spermatogenesis.

Meiosis is illustrated with two pairs of chromosomes for simplicity. Human cells begin meiosis with 23 pairs of chromosomes. In spermatogenesis, 2n indicates diploid cells and n indicates haploid cells.

tetrad. Cross-links are formed and the homologous chromosomes break and exchange parts of their chromatids (Burnet 2003). This exchange of genetic material between homologous chromosomes forms new combinations of genetic material. This is a very important part of meiosis and ensures genetic diversity in the offspring (Baker 1992). No two germ cells are the same.

During metaphase I the spindle apparatus forms and chromosomes become attached to it at the equator. During anaphase I, the two sets of chromosomes separate and move to opposite poles of the cell. Each chromosome from the homologous pair moves in a random way to one of the poles; this random assortment of chromosomes also enhances genetic diversity. At the end of telophase I, the two groups of chromosomes are at opposite ends of the cell. Cytokinesis divides the cytoplasm and two cells form. The cells then enter the second meiotic division. In this division, which is similar to mitosis, the individual chromatids of the chromosomes are separated during anaphase II.

The female reproductive system

The female reproductive system consists of the primary sex organs, the ovaries and the fallopian or uterine tubes, the uterus, vagina and the vulva (see Fig. 9.6). The ovaries are almond-shaped structures that have the same embryonic origin as the testes. The ovary has an outer layer, the cortex, and a deeper section called the medulla. The medulla is composed of fibrous connective tissue containing blood vessels, lymphatic vessels and nerves, whilst the cortex consists of highly dense connective tissue containing the follicles in varying states of development. Each follicle is composed of a developing oocyte surrounded by an outer layer of follicle cells (see Fig. 9.6).

Oogenesis

Oogenesis begins in early fetal development. During oogenesis, meiosis begins, but becomes arrested in the first meiotic prophase. The primary oocyte formed exists as a primordial follicle. There are about 7 million primary oocytes present in the ovaries of a female fetus (Shaw 2001). At birth, all germ cells are arrested in this prophase I stage as primary oocytes. This store of primordial follicles present in the ovary at birth represents the lifetime's supply of developing oocytes. There is no further development until there are raised levels of FSH at puberty.

After puberty, the ovary cycles between a follicular phase (maturing follicles) and a luteal phase (presence of the corpus luteum). The ovarian cycle lasts approximately 28 days. In each ovarian cycle, several primary oocytes are stimulated to proceed through the first meiotic division (see Fig. 9.7). Only one of these proceeds to the mature Graafian follicle stage. The first meiotic division completes prior to ovulation. The secondary oocyte formed is haploid with a single set of chromosomes. The second meiotic division then begins, but becomes locked into metaphase II. Meiosis is only completed at fertilization. At each meiotic division, polar bodies form; these are packets of discarded nuclear material with virtually no cytoplasm. The two meiotic divisions lead to the formation of one ovum with a large amount of cytoplasm.

During the follicular phase, as the primary oocyte matures within a follicle, the follicular cells secrete oestrogen. The mature Graafian follicle bulges on the outer surface of the ovary and at the midpoint of the cycle the secondary oocyte is released from the ovary. Ovulation results from a surge of LH (Shaw 2001). Following ovulation, the luteal phase begins in which the empty follicle forms a corpus luteum that synthesizes progesterone. The secondary oocyte, which was released from the Graafian follicle, passes into the fallopian tube.

The fallopian tube is about 10 cm long and lined with ciliated epithelium. The ovum is transported by the combined efforts of peristalsis and cilia towards the uterus. The uterus has a vascular glandular lining called the endometrium and this is where implantation occurs, following fertilization. At the lower end of the uterus, the cervix connects the uterus to the vagina. The cervix is lined by columnar epithelium containing mucus-secreting cells. Mucous secretions from the cervix vary during the cycle. The secretions become less viscous and more receptive to spermatozoa around the time of ovulation. At other times, the viscous mucus makes it less likely for sperm to enter the uterus and travel to the fallopian tubes. The lining of the vagina is stratified, squamous non-keratinized epithelium.

The place where the two types of epithelium from the cervix and vagina meet is called the squamo-columnar junction. The transformation zone where the two types of epithelial cell merge is the common site of cervical cancer (Cook 1997). Early recognition of pre-cancerous changes occurring in this transformation zone can be achieved by taking a smear of cells for checking in cervical screening (Cook 1997, Desai 1999).

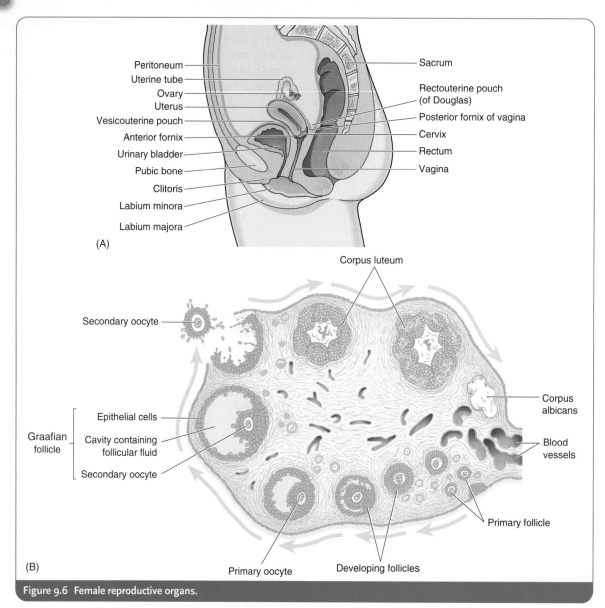

Figure 9.6 Female reproductive organs.

(A) The ovary is the primary sex organ. (B) The diagram of the ovary shows structures that develop during the menstrual cycle. They would not be seen in the ovary at the same time. (Reproduced with kind permission from Waugh & Grant 2001.)

The menstrual cycle

The menstrual cycle begins at puberty and is under the control of hormones from the hypothalamic–pituitary–gonadal axis (HPG axis). Gonadotrophin-releasing hormone (GnRH) from the hypothalamus stimulates the anterior pituitary gland to secrete FSH and LH. FSH stimulates the development of the follicles in the ovary as indicated and LH promotes ovulation and the development of the corpus luteum (see Fig. 9.7). Oestrogen from the follicular cells promotes the healing and repair of the endometrium in the proliferative phase and progesterone from the corpus luteum causes the endometrium to become more glandular in the secretory phase (Aplin 1990). There are three interconnecting cycles in the menstrual cycle: the hormonal cycle, the ovarian cycle and the uterine cycle (see Fig. 9.7).

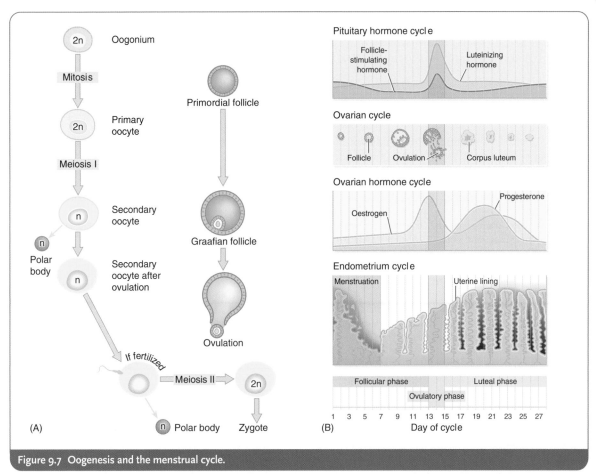

Figure 9.7 Oogenesis and the menstrual cycle.

(A) Oogenesis showing development of the follicle and meiotic divisions. (B) The menstrual cycle showing hormonal cycles, the ovarian cycle and changes in the endometrium.

References

Andrews G R 2001 Promoting health and function in an ageing population. British Medical Journal 322(7288):728–729

Aplin J 1990 The menstrual cycle. Biological Sciences Review 3(2):13–17

Barker D 2001 Cutting edge. THES, 1st June, p 22

Baker T 1992 Meiosis and mammalian gamete formation. Biological Sciences Review 4(4):24–27

Barrowclough D, Ford F 2000 Folic acid fortification. Practical Midwife 3(6):32–33

Bee J 1994 Embryo implantation. Biological Sciences Review 6(4):2–6

Bickmore W 1995 Dance of the chromosomes. MRC News 66:14–18

Bickmore W 1998 Dance of the chromosomes. Biological Sciences Review 11(2):11–14

Bogin B 1999 Patterns of human growth, 2nd edn. Cambridge University Press, Cambridge

Brown B 1998 Telomerase – secret of life. Biological Sciences Review 11(2):28–30

Burnet L 2003 Mechanisms of meiosis. Biological Sciences Review 15(4):20–24

Carr T 1995 Wait for the signal. MRC News 66:19–22

Castronovo V, Kusaki M, Chariot A et al 1994 Homeobox genes: potential candidates for the transcriptional control of the transformed and invasive phenotype. Biochemical Pharmacology 47(1):137–143

Chantler E 2003 Spermatogenesis. Biological Sciences Review 15(4):10–14

Cook R 1997 Cervical screening. Nursing Standard 11(151):40–46

Cooke J 1995 How a cell finds its place in life. MRC News 66:23–27

Desai M 1999 Cervical smear testing. Biological Sciences Review 11(4):38–41

Dudley K 1995 Determinedly male. Biological Sciences Review 7(3):28–31

Duffy C A 2002 Feminine gospels. The map woman. Picador, London, p 3

Evan G I, Vousden K H 2001 Proliferation, cell cycle and apoptosis in cancer. Nature 411(6835):342–348

Evans P 1994 Growth factors. Biological Sciences Review 7(1):18–20

Gepstein L 2002 Derivation and potential applications of human embryonic stem cells. Circulation Research 91(10): 866–876

Green L R 2001 Programming of endocrine mechanisms of cardiovascular control and growth. Journal of the Society for Gynecologic Investigation 8(2):57–68

Green R 1994 Old age. In: Case R M, Waterhouse J M (eds) Human physiology, age, stress, and the environment. Oxford University Press, Oxford, p 99–123

Gordon N 1997 Nutrition and cognitive function. Brain Development 19:165–170

Gull D 1996 Understanding division. Biological Sciences Review 8(5):2–6

Hasenau S, Covington C 2002 Neural tube defects: prevention and folic acid. American Journal of Maternal Child Nursing 27(2):87–91

Herbert R 1991 The normal ageing process reviewed. Nursing Standard 5(51):36–39

Hipkiss A 1994 Why do we age? Biological Sciences Review 6(4):26–29

Hodgson L 1991 Why do we need sleep? Relating theory to nursing practice. Journal of Advances in Nursing 16: 1503–1510

Holloszy J O 2000 The biology of ageing. Mayo Clinic Proceedings 75(Supplement):S3–S9

Hopkin K 1999 Making Methuselah. Scientific American Presents 10(3):32–36

Hyams J 2002 The cell cycle and mitosis. Biological Sciences Review 14(4):37–41

Isley W L 2002 Growth hormone therapy for adults: not ready for prime time? Annals of Internal Medicine 137(3):190–196

Josefson D 2000 Adding fatty acids to baby milk improves development. British Medical Journal 320:735a

Khaw K 1997 Healthy aging. British Medical Journal 315(7115): 1090–1096

Kipling D, Faragher R 1999 Telomeres: ageing hard or hardly ageing? Nature 398(6724):191–193

Kirkwood T 1999 The time of our lives. Weidenfield & Nicolson, London

Kirkwood T 2002 Unravelling the mysteries of human ageing. Biological Sciences Review 14(3):33–37

Kühholzer-Cabot B, Brem G 2002 Aging of animals produced by somatic cell nuclear transfer. Experimental Gerontology 37(12):1317–1323

Laron Z 2001 Insulin-like growth factor 1 (IGF-1): a growth hormone. Molecular Pathology 54(5):311–316

Leese H 1989 Fertilisation. Biological Sciences Review 2(1):2–6

Leonard W R, Robertson M L 1994 Evolutionary perspectives on human nutrition: the influence of brain and body size on diet and metabolism. American Journal of Human Biology 6:77–88

Lithgow G 1998 The biology of ageing. Biological Sciences Review 10(3):18–21

Lucas A 1996 Is future health 'programmed' by infant nutrition? MRC 71:34–37

Meier P, Finch A, Evan G 2000 Apoptosis in development. Nature 407(6805):796–801

Miquel J 2001 Nutrition and ageing. Public Health Nutrition 4(6A):1385–1388

Monk M 1992 The mammalian embryo. Biological Sciences Review 4(3):18–20

Nurse P 1999 To divide or not to divide. Biological Sciences Review 11(4):2–5

Pedersen R A 1999 Embryonic stem cells for medicine. Scientific American Presents 10(3):18–23

Phillips D I W 2002 Endocrine programming and fetal origins of adult disease. Trends in Endocrinology and Metabolism 13(9):363

Polifka J E, Friedman J M 2002 Medical genetics: 1. Clinical teratology in the age of genomics. Canadian Medical Association Journal 167(3):265–273

Raff M 1995 Why are your cells waiting to kill themselves? MRC News 66:28–30

Rubin P 1998 Fortnightly review: drug treatment during pregnancy. British Medical Journal 317(7171):1503–1506

Seaman C 1997 Nutrition in pregnancy: what the papers say. British Journal of Midwifery 9(1):62–63

Shalet S 2000 Growth hormone: the elixir of youth? Biological Sciences Review 12(4):26–28

Sharek P J, Bergman D A 2000 The effect of inhaled steroids on the linear growth of children with asthma: a meta-analysis. Pediatrics 106(1):E8

Shaw H 2001 Menopause. Biological Sciences Review 14(1): 2–6

Simon D, Lucidarme N, Prieir A M et al 2001 Linear growth in children suffering from juvenile idiopathic arthritis requiring steroid therapy: natural history and effects of growth hormone treatment on linear growth. Journal of Pediatrics, Endocrinology and Metabolism 14(Suppl 6): 1483–1486

Sinclair D, Dangerfield P 1998 Human growth after birth. Oxford University Press, Oxford

Small G W 2002 What we need to know about age related memory loss. British Medical Journal 324(7352):1502–1505

Spencer N J, Logan S 2002 The treatment of parental height as a biological factor in studies of birth weight and childhood growth. Archives of Disease in Childhood 87(3):184–187

Stanworth S J, Newland A C 2001 Stem cells: progress in research and edging towards the clinical setting. Clinical Medicine 1(5):378–382

Turner A 2001 Essential fatty acids for maternal and fetal nutrition. British Journal of Midwifery 9(1):62–63

Untergasser G, Rumpold H, Hermann M et al 1999 Proliferative disorders of the aging human prostate: involvement of protein hormones and their receptors. Experimental Gerontology 34(2):275–287

Van Cauter E, Plat L 1996 Physiology of growth hormone secretion during sleep. Journal of Pediatrics 128(5 Part 2):S32–S37

Voss L D 1999 Short but normal. Archives of Disease in Childhood 81(4):370–371

Walker J 1994 The power behind the cell. MRC News 64:10–13

Wallace D C 1999 Mitochondrial diseases in mouse and man. Science 283:1482–1488

Wallis G A 1997 Getting to grips with hand development. Biological Sciences Review 10(2):33–37

Waugh A, Grant A 2001 Ross and Wilson: Anatomy and physiology in health and illness. Churchill Livingstone, Edinburgh

Williams N 2002 Dolly clouds cloning hopes. Current Biology 12(3):R79–R80

10

GENETICS

'Although genetics is all about inheritance, inheritance is certainly not all about genetics. Nearly all inherited characteristics more complicated than a single change in the DNA involve gene and environment acting together.'

(Jones 1993)

The ability to grow and develop from a fertilized egg into a fully functioning adult human being is utterly dependent on an individual's genes. Genes are passed from parents to their children via the egg and sperm at conception. The instructions to make a human being are written in these genes. The whole set of instructions is contained within about 35 000 genes in the nuclei of our cells (Middleton & Peters 2001). These genes are responsible for directing the development of the structure of the body and its tissues and organs, and how the body and its component parts function.

Genes play a fundamental role in health and disease and an understanding of the principles of inheritance is therefore becoming increasingly important. Genetics is the study of the patterns of inheritance. The complete set of genetic information held in each nucleus is called the genome. Genes are composed of deoxyribonucleic acid (DNA) and contain instructions for the manufacture of proteins. Chromosomes consist of two identical chromatids, each a single DNA molecule coiled up with proteins (see Fig. 10.1).

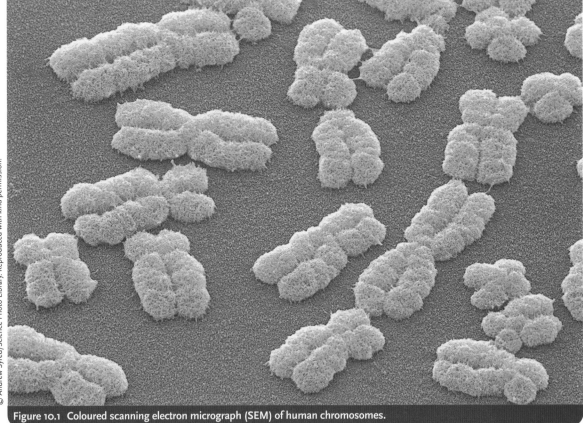

Figure 10.1 Coloured scanning electron micrograph (SEM) of human chromosomes.

Each chromosome comprises two chromatids joined at the centromere.

Each cell apart from the gametes has 23 pairs of chromosomes, which become visible during cell division (see Ch. 9). There are 22 pairs of autosomes with one chromosome in each homologous pair inherited from each parent. The 23rd pair of sex chromosomes is two X chromosomes for a female and an X and Y chromosome for a male.

Deoxyribonucleic acid

In 1869, a Swiss biochemist, Miescher, discovered that all living cells contained the same substance in their nuclei. This substance was known later as nucleic acid and in the 1920s deoxyribonucleic acid (DNA) and ribonucleic acid (RNA) were identified (Porter 1997).

Understanding the structure of DNA, deduced by Watson and Crick in 1953, was essential to the breakthrough in comprehending how genetic information passed from parents to offspring (Lewis & Grant 2002). Originally it was the proteins associated with DNA in the chromosomes that were thought to be transmitting inherited characteristics, but once the structure of DNA was known it was established that DNA was the hereditary material, the 'genetic blueprint'.

The double helical structure of DNA is well known, although this feature is irrelevant in its ability to code information. The two side chains of the double helix are made up of sugars and phosphates. The sugar in DNA is deoxyribose and with phosphate forms the 'backbone' of DNA. The two strands of the DNA are linked together with bases acting like the rungs of a ladder. Each sugar–phosphate–base unit is called a nucleotide, and many join together to make up each strand. The bases are adenine (A), thymine (T), guanine (G) and cytosine (C). The shapes and dimensions of the bases dictate the way in which they link or pair up. In order to form a double stranded molecule with a regular structure, A always pairs with T and G always pairs with C – this is known as base pairing. The base pairs are joined by weak bonds that allow the strands to be easily separated so that they can be copied prior to cell division (see Fig. 10.2).

In the previous chapter, the concept of equal and exact copies of the DNA being divided between two daughter cells during cell division was introduced. The remarkable ability to self-replicate prior to cell division is one of the two key functions of DNA; the other function is to store coded instructions for living (Lehman 1991). DNA is replicated in the S phase of the cell cycle (see p. 112) and when the cell divides each of the two daughter cells receives identical genetic information to the parent cell.

Replication of DNA

The double-stranded structure of DNA facilitates the mechanism for replication since each strand can act as a template for the two 'daughter' strands. The first stage is for the two strands to separate and unwind, rather like unzipping a zip. A new strand of DNA forms as an enzyme, DNA polymerase, adds the correct nucleotides from an abundant supply within the nucleus. The obligatory base pairing ensures two identical DNA molecules form; each half of the original DNA molecule has duplicated itself to form a new DNA molecule (see Fig. 10.2). Groups of enzymes move along the DNA molecule searching for any errors. Wrong nucleotides in sections of DNA are noticed as distortions and corrected (Lehman 1991). Repairs are made to the DNA molecule by appropriate enzymes; if these repairs are overlooked then mutations can occur (Kang 2002).

Genetic code

Genes direct the manufacture, or synthesis, of all the body's proteins (Lewis & Grant 2002). The functional and structural roles of proteins dictate what the cell does and how it functions. Proteins are crucial molecules in many respects (see Ch. 3); it is our proteins that shape our growth and development into unique individuals. There are 20 amino acids, and these link up in a multitude of ways to create the vast array of human proteins.

The concept that the amino acid sequence is crucial to the shape and function of proteins was introduced in Chapter 3. In the assembly of proteins and polypeptides, amino acids are linked correctly due to the instructions contained in the sequence of bases in the DNA molecule. Each gene is a DNA sequence made up of a series of 'codons' that codes for a protein or polypeptide. Three nucleotides make up a triplet or codon, and each codon specifies a particular amino acid. The series of codons in a gene carries instructions to assemble amino acids in the right sequence to make a particular protein (Bulleid 2001) (see Fig. 10.3).

During protein synthesis the coded information in DNA is transcribed to a messenger RNA molecule (mRNA). There are four bases or letters in the code within DNA and mRNA and, because there are three

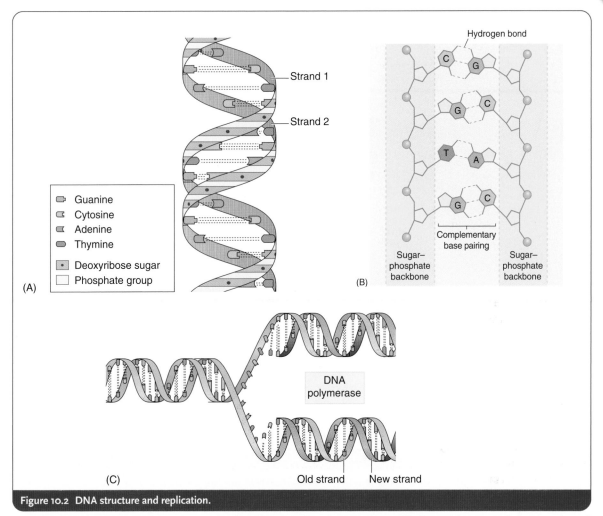

Figure 10.2 **DNA structure and replication.**

(A) Deoxyribonucleic acid (DNA). (B) DNA structure showing complementary pairing of the bases. (C) DNA replication is achieved by unwinding of the double helix and DNA polymerase adding new bases. (Part (A) reproduced with kind permission from Waugh & Grant 2001.)

bases in each codon, there are 4^3 or 64 different codon combinations. This means there are more than enough different codons to represent each of the 20 amino acids. Some of the extra permutations are for stop codons that note the end of the mRNA sequence for a particular protein, and some amino acids are represented by more than one codon (O'Keefe 2003).

Protein synthesis

There are two stages in the manufacture of proteins. The first stage is transcription and involves the information coded in the DNA sequence being copied into another nucleic acid called messenger RNA (mRNA). The mRNA leaves the nucleus via the nuclear pores and enters the cytoplasm, where protein synthesis occurs in a process called translation. The sequence of bases in the RNA dictates the building of a protein with the correct amino acid sequence.

The first step in transcription is the unwinding of the DNA sequence coding for the protein. The abundant free nucleotides in the nucleus align themselves correctly opposite the DNA sequence with the help of an enzyme, RNA polymerase. A single-stranded mRNA molecule is formed that is literally a copy of the DNA template. In mRNA, the base uracil (U) replaces thymine (T). The bases in the DNA sequence dictate the sequence of nucleotides that link up to form the mRNA

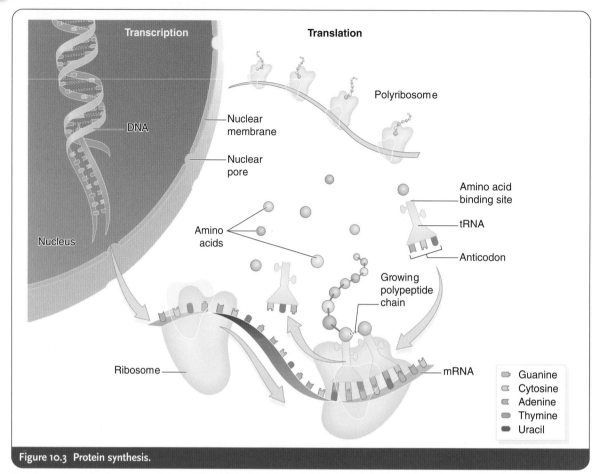

Figure 10.3 Protein synthesis.

Protein synthesis involves transcription of the code in DNA to messenger RNA (mRNA) and translation of this message into the correct sequence of amino acids linked together in a protein.

molecule. The base pairing is that U and A always pair up and C and G form a pair (as in DNA). The mRNA molecule then unzips from the DNA template and diffuses into the cytoplasm (Bulleid 1992).

Protein synthesis takes place in ribosomes, small bodies constructed out of ribosomal RNA and proteins (Bulleid 1992), which are often associated with rough endoplasmic reticulum (see p. 6). During translation, several ribosomes will read the code in the mRNA molecule at the same time. Each ribosome synthesizes a protein molecule by linking amino acids in the right sequence at the rate of about 40 amino acids per second (Bulleid 1992).

The correct sequencing of amino acids in the assembly of proteins is ensured by another RNA molecule called transfer RNA (tRNA). tRNA molecules are able to link up with specific amino acids from the cytoplasm. tRNA is a single-stranded RNA molecule that doubles back on itself to form double-stranded sections

and a number of loops. One of the loops contains the anticodon, a triplet of bases that are complementary to the codon on the mRNA molecule. The non-loop end attaches the appropriate amino acid. Each type of amino acid has its own tRNA molecule with its unique specific anticodon (O'Keefe 2003). As the ribosome reads the code, it translates each codon and the tRNA molecule deposits or 'transfers' the right amino acid to the elongating polypeptide chain (see Fig. 10.3).

Gene expression

The important role of genes in growth and development was introduced in Chapter 9. A group of genes fundamental in directing development and differentiation called homeobox genes were highlighted (see p. 116) (Castronovo et al 1994) because they control the pattern of expression of other genes during development (Wallis 1997). Gene expression is central to the variety of cells in the human body. Every cell has the potential to express all its genes, but in reality only expresses a very small number at any time. Differences between cells are attributable to the different proteins they contain and this in turn depends on which genes are expressed (McLennan 1994). The switching on and off of genes is complex and tightly controlled; problems occurring in the signalling processes controlling gene expression are associated with cancer (McLennan 1994).

A number of regulatory DNA sequences are associated with genes (Lewis & Grant 2002) which have to be activated by transcription factors (or gene regulatory products) before the gene is switched on and transcription begins. The regulation of gene expression is necessarily complex and involves the interaction of a number of factors (McLennan 1994).

Human genome map

Characteristics such as hair colour, height and body build are shaped by the genes we have inherited from our parents. Genes also make us more likely to develop some diseases and not others. The human genome project has produced a map showing the location of genes on human chromosomes (Collins et al 2003). The information is like a giant directory or 'handbook of human life' (Coghlan 2000). Knowing the location and identity of all human genes will enhance the possibility of predicting the occurrence of genetic diseases and determining the genetic basis of diseases. However, bridging the gap between discovering the genes that predispose an individual to develop a particular disease and being able to intervene or help in the prevention and management of certain diseases remains formidable (Kent 1999). In addition to the huge technical difficulties still to be overcome, there are many ethico-legal and social implications associated with the knowledge and techniques of molecular genetics that need to be discussed and critically analysed prior to policy making (Mendelsohn 1999, Collins et al 2003).

Genes and inheritance

The roots of our present understanding of genetics and disease come from the work of Gregor Mendel, a monk who studied the inheritance of characteristics in pea plants. Mendel outlined patterns of inheritance even before genes were described. Mendelian inheritance applies to characteristics and conditions that are inherited from either or both parents in one or two pairs of genes in patterns called autosomal dominant, recessive or X-linked inheritance.

In addition to Mendelian inheritance patterns, characteristics such as height and most common diseases including heart disease, cancer, asthma, diabetes and some forms of mental illness result from the interaction of many genes (polygenes) with environmental factors; this is called multifactorial inheritance (Peters et al 2001). Another category of genetic conditions involves the chromosomes; chromosome anomalies are due to a change in the usual number (aneuploidy) or a structural change (Middleton & Peters 2001).

Single gene disorders are due to mutations in either one or both members of the gene pair or to mutations in genes on the X chromosome. Mutations are due to the loss or gain of DNA (length mutations) or to a change in the genetic code of the DNA sequence. The latter are point mutations and are due to a single nucleotide base being exchanged for a different one. Gene mutations lead to a change in the form and function of the proteins they code for with varying effects on cell function and health.

Each gene occupies a particular position (locus) on a chromosome; the genes that occupy the same locus on homologous chromosomes are called alleles. One allele from each pair originates from the mother and the other one from the father. The combinations of genes that an individual has are known as the genotype whilst the phenotype describes the characteristics the individual possesses. When an individual has two alleles that are the same they are described as homozygous; when the alleles are different, the individual is said to be heterozygous.

Autosomal dominant single gene conditions

Examples of autosomal dominant diseases include Huntington's disease, neurofibromatosis and polyposis coli (Middleton & Peters 2001). Huntington's disease is a late onset degenerative disease of the brain. The gene associated with Huntington's disease, the huntingtin variant gene, contains a triplet of bases, cytosine, adenine and guanine (CAG), repeated in a stretch many times. In the usual huntingtin gene the CAG triplet is repeated somewhere between 9 and 35 times (Cattaneo et al 2002), but in individuals with the huntingtin variant gene, the CAG triplet is repeated between 40 and 60 times. The protein encoded for by the variant gene has a mutated structure; the CAG triplet codes for the amino acid glutamine and with many extra copies of this amino acid the protein becomes dysfunctional. The altered protein seems to interact differently with other proteins causing unusual protein aggregates to form. These are toxic and lead to dysfunction and ultimately death of brain cells (Cattaneo et al 2002).

In autosomal dominant inheritance, both males and females can have the condition. Individuals in each generation are affected and the condition can be transmitted by both sexes to either male or female offspring. Family pedigrees are constructed to show the pattern of inheritance (see Fig. 10.4). Genetic diagrams illustrate the inheritance of single genes. The expressed gene is the dominant allele and is usually represented by a capital letter whilst the gene that is not expressed is the recessive allele and is denoted by a lower case letter (see Fig. 10.4). When one parent has the gene variant for Huntington's disease the expected ratio of affected to unaffected offspring is 50:50. This means that every child has a 1 in 2 chance of inheriting the huntingtin gene variant and developing Huntington's disease later in life.

Autosomal recessive single gene conditions

There are many different autosomal recessive traits in humans, including cystic fibrosis, phenylketonuria and sickle cell disease. The incidence of phenylketonuria (PKU) is about 1 in 14 000 (Simpson et al 1997, Kwon & Farrell 2000). It is caused by mutations in a gene on chromosome 12, encoding an enzyme that converts phenylalanine (an amino acid) into tyrosine. Deficiency of this enzyme results in an accumulation of phenylalanine and its metabolites, which are toxic to the brain. There are many different mutations that have variable effects on enzyme activity (Tyfield 1997). To prevent neurological damage, infants and children with phenylketonuria consume a restricted diet with low levels of phenylalanine supplemented with an artificial amino mixture containing vitamins and minerals (Clark 1992). When a child has an autosomal recessive disease it means that both parents were heterozygous carriers of the recessive variant gene. The probability of these parents having a child with phenylketonuria is 1 in 4 (see Fig. 10.4).

The most frequently inherited disease in Britain is cystic fibrosis (Nurse 1992). The incidence of babies born with cystic fibrosis is about 1 in 2000 in the UK (Brock et al 1998, Cunningham & Marshall 1998). This disease is characterized by the production of viscous mucus, which in the lungs leads to frequent chest infections. Thick secretions also block the pancreatic duct and prevent pancreatic enzymes reaching the duodenum to digest food. Management of an individual with cystic fibrosis includes physiotherapy to loosen lung secretions, antibiotics to prevent infection and replacement enzyme tablets to avoid the consequences of malnutrition resulting from the impaired digestion (Doull 2001).

The gene involved in cystic fibrosis encodes a protein involved in the transport of chloride ions across epithelial cell membranes (Read 1992). Everyone has two copies of this gene, one from each parent located on each copy of chromosome 7. Because cystic fibrosis is a recessive disease only individuals who have inherited the cystic fibrosis variant gene from both parents are affected with the condition. Most of the mutations of this gene result from a deletion of three nucleotides in the DNA sequence meaning that the chloride transport protein has one amino acid missing (Read 1992). This results in a dysfunctional protein with serious consequences for the transport of chloride ions across cell membranes. The frequency of the cystic fibrosis gene variant in the UK population is about 1 in 20 (Cunningham & Marshall 1998). Individuals with this gene variant are carriers and have no symptoms.

Individuals with sickle cell disease (see p. 32) inherit two variant β globin genes that code for sickle haemoglobin (HbS) (see Ch. 3 to remind you of the globin chains found in the haemoglobin molecule). When oxygen levels are low, HbS changes structure and distorts the red blood cell, transforming it into a sickle shape. Individuals who have just one of the HbS variant β globin genes have an increased protection against malaria. There is a point mutation in the β globin gene found on chromosome 11 and this results in sickle haemoglobin in which just one amino acid is different from HbA (Grant 1997). Heterozygous individuals with sickle cell trait rarely have symptoms, although may exhibit a very mild form of anaemia in some circumstances. This implies that both alleles are expressed in an individual with sickle cell trait producing HbA and HbS. Since neither allele is completely dominant it illustrates that there are exceptions to mendelian inheritance patterns (Jones 1993).

X-linked recessive single gene conditions

In this pattern of inheritance, the altered gene is found on the X chromosome, which has other genes apart from those that determine female sex. Females have two X chromosomes whilst men only have one. This means that any mutant recessive genes on the X chromosome will be expressed in men because there is only

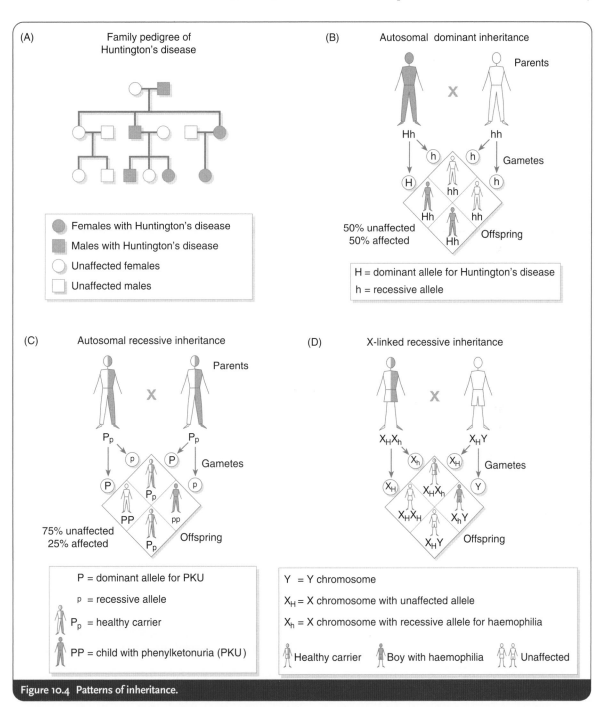

Figure 10.4 Patterns of inheritance.

(A) Family pedigree showing the inheritance of Huntington's disease. (B) Genetic diagram showing autosomal dominant inheritance of Huntington's disease. (C) Genetic diagram illustrating autosomal recessive inheritance of phenylketonuria. (D) Genetic diagram demonstrating X-linked recessive inheritance of haemophilia.

one copy of the gene, whilst in females the unaltered, working dominant allele on the second X chromosome will be expressed.

Haemophilia, Duchenne muscular dystrophy and red–green colour blindness are examples of conditions caused by recessive alleles located on the X chromosome that preferentially affect males. Haemophilia results in the deficiency of one of the blood clotting factors, Factor VIII or Factor IX, which leads to variable effects on blood coagulation (Susman-Shaw & Harrington 1999). Sons born to a heterozygous mother (carrier) have an equal chance of inheriting the X chromosome with the haemophilia gene or the unaffected X chromosome. This means they have a 50% or 1 in 2 chance of having haemophilia (see Fig. 10.4). The mutations causing haemophilia are very diverse and include point mutations, deletions and inversions. Point mutations are most common and are due to a change in one amino acid within either of the proteins, Factor VIII or Factor IX (Bowen 2002).

Not only do individual genes contribute to genetic diseases, but whole or parts of chromosomes that contain many genes are also involved. Chromosome disorders can result from an abnormal number of chromosomes or from changes in chromosome structure.

Chromosomal disorders

Down syndrome is the most common chromosome disorder in live born infants and most often results from inheriting an extra chromosome 21 at conception. This is the result of an error occurring in meiosis (see p. 120). If the chromosomes fail to separate (non-disjunction) during the first meiotic division, one of the daughter cells will have 24 chromosomes and the other one will have 22. When a gamete with 24 chromosomes joins one with 23 chromosomes at conception, the zygote has 47 chromosomes. The inheritance of three copies of a chromosome is called a trisomy. The most common cause of trisomy is due to an unequal separation of chromosomes in the first meiotic division in the production of ova (see p. 120) (Burnet 2003).

Most embryos with chromosomes missing or with an additional chromosome are spontaneously aborted. Embryos with trisomy 13, 18 and 21 can develop until full term, although with the exception of trisomy 21, the babies do not usually survive (Burnet 2003).

The risk of having a child with trisomy 21 increases with maternal age which is why women over 35 are offered prenatal diagnosis (Newman 1999). There are many procedures used in genetic testing and screening for genetic and chromosome disorders including ultrasound scanning, amniocentesis, chorionic villi sampling (CVS) and maternal blood screening (Bozzette 2002, Newman 1999). In amniocentesis, a sample of amniotic fluid containing fetal cells is taken for investigation via a needle which crosses the abdomen into the amniotic sac inside the uterus. Chorionic villus sampling involves removing trophoblastic villi from the chorionic sac. In both these procedures, karyotyping is performed which enables chromosomes to be visualized and trisomies or translocations detected (Bozzette 2002). There are many ethical issues to consider in prenatal testing and screening and the Human Fertilisation and Embryology Authority (HEFA) is an important body that monitors and regulates new advances (Newman 1999).

Children and adults with Down syndrome exhibit a broad range of learning abilities and disabilities together with an increased likelihood of heart defects, increased risk of infection and premature ageing (Dewhurst 1998). It is now known that there are three types of Down syndrome: trisomy 21, translocation and mosaicism. Trisomy 21 is most frequent, accounting for 95% of cases. In about 4% of cases, Down syndrome results from the translocation of a part of chromosome 21 to another chromosome. This is most often chromosome 14 (Dewhurst 1998). This means that cells have two copies of the chromosome 21 and an extra part of chromosome 21 in every cell. Mosaicism occurs rarely and results in some cells containing 46 chromosomes whilst others have 47 chromosomes. This means that the extra chromosome 21 has arisen during a mitotic division in the early embryo. As the cells continue to divide some will have the usual number of chromosomes and others will have trisomy 21 (Dewhurst 1998).

Multifactorial inheritance

Most human characteristics and common diseases such as heart disease, diabetes and cancer are thought to result from the complex interaction of many genes, lifestyle and other environmental factors (Middleton & Peters 2001, Peters et al 2001). An individual inherits

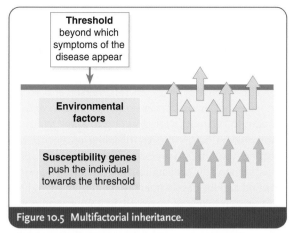

Figure 10.5 Multifactorial inheritance.

Lifestyle and other environmental factors interact with polygenes and push the individual over the threshold so they have the disease.

many genes (polygenes) that predispose them to certain characteristics or diseases. The cumulative effect of a group of polygenes and their interactions increases an individual's susceptibility to a particular disease or diseases. The likelihood of developing the disease is further enhanced through a subtle interplay with certain environmental factors (Coghlan 2000).

A collection of particular genes may cause the individual to approach a critical 'threshold' and the specific environmental influences may push the individual over the critical threshold so that they develop the disease (see Fig. 10.5). The heritability of a condition gives an estimate of the genetic contribution resulting from the complex interplay of many genes (Sanders & Gejman 2001).

Asthma

The aetiology of asthma, the most predominant chronic disease in children in developed countries, is multifactorial (Cookson 2002). The heritability of asthma is estimated to be 68% in one study of four-year-old twins (Koeppen-Schomerus et al 2001). Many genes have been identified that contribute towards an individual's susceptibility to asthma, the most significant on chromosomes 5, 6, 12 and 13 (Cookson 2002). The incidence of asthma is increasing, but since genes cannot spread through populations at a rate that could account for the increase in asthma, other factors must be responsible (Hamilton 1998). A lack of exposure to dirt and childhood infections may be influential in causing the immune system to respond inappropriately to allergens (Hamilton 1998). Allergens such as pollens, animal

dander and house mites provoke bronchial constriction, excess mucus production and inflammation, which result in the familiar symptoms of wheezing and shortness of breath (Renauld 2001). Stress is also thought to contribute to asthma morbidity in complex ways (see p. 73) (Wright et al 1998). Individuals inherit a number of genes that increase their susceptibility to asthma; if they are then exposed to certain combinations of lifestyle and other environmental factors they develop the disease.

Schizophrenia

Schizophrenia affects about 1% of the population worldwide and is characterized by major disturbances in thinking, perception, mood and behaviour. The genetic contribution to schizophrenia is not clear, although both genetic and environmental factors are considered to play a role in the aetiology of schizophrenia (Sanders & Gejman 2001). The history of genes and schizophrenia is not a happy one since the spurious belief that schizophrenia was genetically transmitted led to the eugenic sterilization of individuals with schizophrenia by Nazi geneticists and psychiatrists (Rose et al 1984). Evidence for heritability in schizophrenia comes from twin, family and adoption studies and these tend to support the view that several to many genes are involved (Gottesman & Shields 1982, Sanders & Gejman 2001). However, the findings of these studies and their interpretations are controversial (Rose et al 1984, Breggin 1993). Heritability is estimated to be between 60–80% in a number of studies (Kendler 2001). Current thinking is that susceptibility genes together with social and cultural factors push some people towards exhibiting schizophrenic symptoms. A number of genes that might confer susceptibility to schizophrenia have been identified (Levinson et al 2000, Bassett et al 2002). The identification of these genes and their products together with a greater understanding of environmental factors which interact with these genes may lead to advances in the management of schizophrenia (Sanders & Gejman 2001).

Cancer genetics

Cancer describes a set of diseases in which the growth and division of normal cells is disrupted. The development of cancer (carcinogenesis) is multifactorial and involves a number of steps all of which involve gene alterations (Peters et al 2001).

Cancer cells result from mutations in the sequence of nucleotides in the DNA of genes controlling cell growth and division. A single cell usually has mutations in several different genes before it becomes cancerous, and these mutations accumulate a long time before any physiological change is detected (Itzhaki 1999).

Mutations in DNA may be either germline (inherited) or somatic (acquired during life) (Cummings & Bingham 1998). An individual who inherits a mutation in a cancer susceptibility gene is one step closer to developing cancer since every cell has the mutation (Peters et al 2001). Cancer-causing (mutagenic) agents in the environment impact on the DNA in our cells thousands of times a day. Mutations in three to seven genes are thought to be necessary in order to transform cells. As cells age they acquire more mutations, which is why the incidence of cancer increases with age (Itzhaki 1999).

There are two classes of genes that play a major role in carcinogenesis; these are the oncogenes and tumour-suppressor genes (Balkwill 1998). Oncogenes code for proteins involved in signalling cells to divide. These aberrant signals enable cells to divide in an uncontrolled fashion. Oncogenes are mutations of a class of genes called proto-oncogenes that code for proteins such as growth factors and receptor proteins in the growth-signalling pathway. Most proto-oncogene mutations occur at a somatic level and cause sporadic cancers. Mutations in proto-oncogenes are dominant and damage to one proto-oncogene leads to an oncogene capable of predisposing the individual to cancer (Balkwill 1998).

Tumour-suppressor genes are present in normal cells and restrain cell proliferation. When they are missing or mutated they enable cells to proliferate in an unregulated fashion leading to tumour growth (Peters et al 2001). Mutations in tumour suppressor genes are recessive which means that both copies of the gene must mutate before cell growth is disrupted (Balkwill 1998).

The p53 gene is probably the most important tumour-suppressor gene and is damaged in about 40% of all cancers (Balkwill 1998). The p53 protein that the gene codes for plays a key role in a cell cycle checkpoint monitoring damage in DNA (see p. 113) (Peters et al 2001). If the p53 gene mutates, its protein product is no longer able to exert control, and a cell with damaged DNA can carry on dividing and copying its damaged DNA (Balkwill 1998).

A further group of genes with a more indirect role in cancer growth have been proposed. These are DNA repair genes and they are involved in maintaining the integrity of the genome in the face of DNA damaging agents, such as ionizing irradiation. Mutations in these genes allow DNA damage to accumulate, increasing the susceptibility to cancer (Itzhaki 1999).

Breast cancer

Breast cancer is the most common cancer in women, with a prevalence of nearly 2% (McPherson et al 2000). Most cases of breast cancer occur sporadically and are thought to be multifactorial in origin. Many genes are implicated in breast cancer including oncogenes and mutated tumour suppressor genes. Gene mutations occur sequentially contributing to a cascade of disrupted function and the development of the cancer. An individual's susceptibility is increased by the inheritance of many genes whose effects are additive, illustrating the polygenic origin of many breast cancers (Lewis 2003).

About 10% of breast cancers are inherited and, of these, inherited mutations in BRCA1 and BRCA2 genes are responsible for about half the cases (Venkitaraman 1999). The inheritance of one of these mutated genes predisposes an individual to develop breast cancer. Both genes are thought to play a role in DNA repair (Venkitaraman 1999, Lewis 2003). Mutations in these genes leads to the disruption in the DNA repair machinery.

A number of environmental factors that interact with susceptibility genes in sporadic breast cancers have been studied, including infections, diet, oestrogens and other hormones (see p. 51) (Cummings & Bingham 1998, McPherson et al 2000, Lawson & Rawlinson 2001). Stress may also be implicated in breast cancer (see p. 76).

Lung cancer

Lung cancer is the most common cause of cancer in developed countries. It is a multifactorial disease resulting from the interaction of polygenes and environmental factors (Kiyohara et al 2002). Genetic susceptibility to lung cancer is suggested in the familial clustering of the disease and the variable influence of lifetime smoking. One in ten lifetime smokers develop lung cancer, suggesting that they have genetic factors that are particularly sensitive to cigarette smoking (Sethi 2002). Some individuals, due to their inheritance of certain genes, are more susceptible to low levels of exposure to carcinogens in cigarette smoke than others (Kiyohara et al 2002). Many genetic factors are responsible for an individual smoker's susceptibility to lung cancer and many chemicals in cigarette smoke are carcinogenic (Hecht 2002). Lung cancer is due to the chronic exposure of DNA in the lungs to carcinogens. Whilst smoking cessation is the most effective way to reduce the likelihood of lung cancer, a knowledge of and ability to screen for genetic susceptibility factors may play a key role in future prevention strategies (Hecht 2002).

It is implicit in the foregoing discussion that an understanding of the DNA variation in the human genome will enable developments in prevention, diagnosis and treatment to occur. Technical advances make it possible to clone animals (Cohen 1998) and to replace gene mutations in gene therapy (Hanak 1998). Information from the human genome project will offer insights into which characteristics are inherited and which are acquired and help to delineate the interplay between genes and the environment in the pathogenesis of certain diseases (Subramanian et al 2001). However, since the majority of common human diseases result from many genes interacting with each other and environmental factors, unravelling the contributions of genes will be immensely challenging (Middleton & Peters 2001, Subramanian et al 2001). There are many pitfalls in this era of molecular medicine, including the potential to diagnose and treat diseases even before they develop clinical manifestations. This knowledge in ill-advised hands could be used to prevent individuals from gaining employment or insurance coverage; and an individual's knowledge of their genetic susceptibility to disease may create anxiety about possible future illness (Gerling et al 2003). Parents will face difficult decisions about prenatal tests and their results (Newman 1999). A key concept that should always be kept at the forefront in this burgeoning field is that the genotype does not exclusively determine the phenotype (Rose et al 1984, Scriver 2002).

Introducing the respiratory system

The role of genes in a number of diseases affecting the respiratory system, including asthma, cystic fibrosis and lung cancer, have been introduced in this chapter, so this is an appropriate place to introduce the respiratory system.

The key role of the respiratory system is to maintain the right amounts of oxygen and carbon dioxide in the internal environment. The respiratory system comprises the lungs and a system of airways that connect the lungs to the external environment. The lungs lie on either side of the heart within the thorax, a cavity separated from the abdomen by the diaphragm, a sheet of muscle involved in breathing.

Form and function of the respiratory tract

Air is drawn into the nose through the nostrils and enters the nasal cavity. The mucous membrane which lines the nasal cavity covers a large surface area and consists of ciliated pseudostratified columnar epithelium containing many mucus-secreting goblet cells (see Fig. 10.6). This epithelium lies over the surface of areolar tissue containing an extensive network of blood capillaries. As air passes through the nasal cavity, heat radiating from the blood warms the air. Evaporation of water from the mucous membrane moistens or humidifies the air and the sticky mucus traps dust and other small particles. Cilia waft the layer of mucus to the pharynx where it is swallowed and any microorganisms are destroyed in the stomach by acidic gastric juice. This filtering process prevents particles reaching the lungs and helps prevent respiratory infections.

Air enters the pharynx at the back of the mouth and passes into the larynx (the voice box) through a small hole called the glottis. This is guarded by the epiglottis, which is a small flap that prevents food entering into the air passages. The larynx contains the vocal cords, which vibrate as air is forced through the larynx when you breathe out.

The trachea is the first part of the bronchial tree, a system of tubes that get smaller as they lead to the alveoli of the lungs. The trachea is a large cylindrical tube that contains C-shaped cartilage rings to prevent the walls collapsing. This ensures that the flow of air in and out of the lungs is always unimpeded. The soft tissue at the back of the trachea enables food to move down the oesophagus. The ciliated epithelial lining of the trachea is similar to that in the nasal cavity and continues to filter air and trap particles.

Cigarette smoking has a number of effects on the bronchial epithelium, including the loss of cilia and proliferation of certain neuroendocrine cells that are important in the regulation of growth and differentiation (Johnson et al 1997). Lung cancer is strongly associated with smoking and there are at least 60 established carcinogens in cigarette smoke. These gradually disrupt DNA and genes that are crucial in control mechanisms, including cell cycle regulation (Hecht 2002).

The trachea divides into the right and left primary bronchi and within each lung the bronchus splits into many branches forming the bronchial tree. C-shaped rings of cartilage are replaced by cartilaginous plates in the bronchi. The amount of cartilage decreases and finally disappears so that cartilage is absent in the bronchioles. The walls of bronchioles contain smooth muscle,

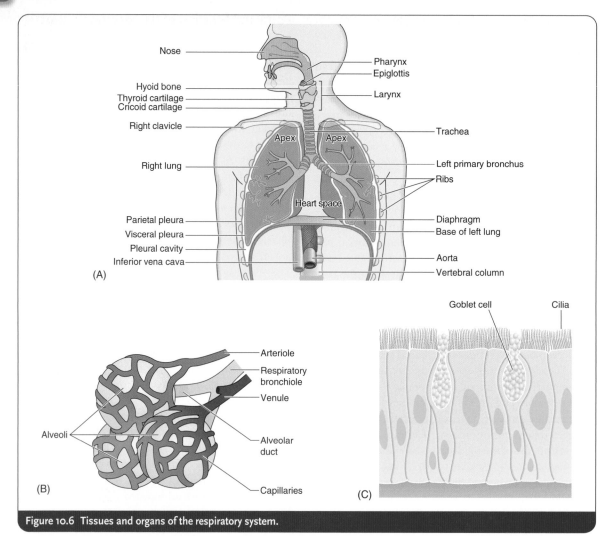

Figure 10.6 Tissues and organs of the respiratory system.

(A) Organs of the respiratory system. (B) Clusters of alveoli and their blood supply. (C) Ciliated pseudostratified columnar epithelium found lining the nasal cavity, trachea, larynx and bronchi. (Parts (A) and (B) reproduced with kind permission from Waugh & Grant 2001.)

which can contract or relax, enabling the bronchioles to constrict or dilate according to physiological needs. In asthma, the bronchial mucosae become swollen, mucus production becomes excessive and the smooth muscle constricts during a hypersensitivity reaction to an allergen (Renauld 2001).

Each bronchiole leads to a bunch of sacs called alveoli surrounded by a dense network of blood capillaries. Alveolar air is separated from the blood by a very thin respiratory membrane (see Fig. 10.7). Gas exchange takes place across this membrane, oxygen diffuses into the blood and carbon dioxide diffuses from blood into the alveoli. The respiratory membrane is well adapted

to gas exchange because it has a very large surface area and is extremely thin. Surfactant, an oily substance composed of phospholipids and proteins, is secreted by type 2 alveolar cells. The thin layer of surfactant covering the alveolar epithelium reduces surface tension (McCormack 1997). This prevents the alveoli from collapsing and sticking shut as air flows in and out during breathing.

Ventilation

Inside the thorax there are two pleural membranes, one lines the inside of the thorax and the other covers the

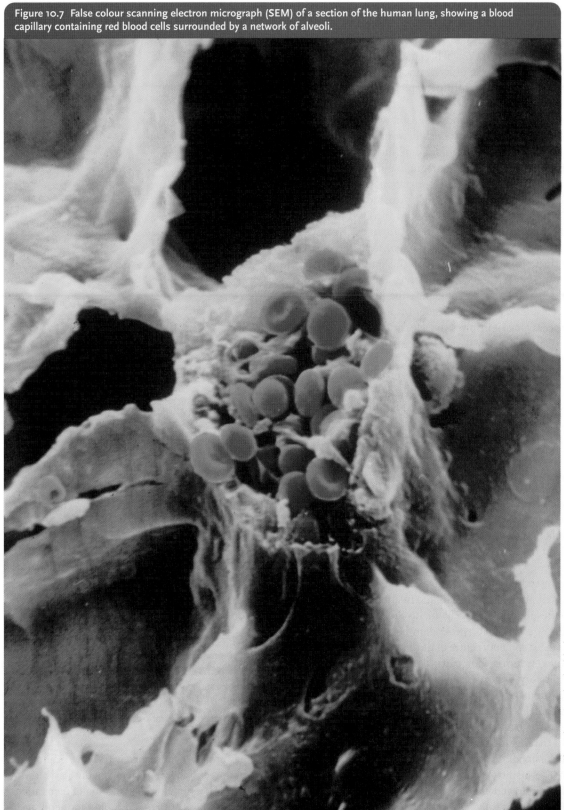

Figure 10.7 False colour scanning electron micrograph (SEM) of a section of the human lung, showing a blood capillary containing red blood cells surrounded by a network of alveoli.

outside of the lungs. The space in between contains a small amount of fluid, which enables the membranes to slide over each other, but not apart (Blanchflower 2002). This cohesion between the two moist pleura enables the lungs to expand, since as the thorax moves up and outwards during inspiration the lungs are stretched along too.

Pulmonary ventilation, or breathing, is the process by which gases are exchanged between the lungs and atmosphere. Breathing is accomplished by movements of the chest wall and diaphragm that inflate and deflate the lungs. Inspiration and expiration movements are accompanied by changes in the size of the thoracic cavity.

In inspiration the key muscles involved in breathing, the diaphragm and external intercostal muscles, contract. This causes the diaphragm to flatten and the thoracic cage to move upward and outward (see Fig. 10.8). The increased volume creates a negative pressure and air rushes in to equilibrate the pressure with the atmospheric pressure outside. Inspiration is an active process since it involves muscle contraction.

Expiration is a passive process in which the diaphragm relaxes and resumes its dome shape and the external intercostal muscles relax, enabling the thoracic cage to move downwards and inwards. This reduces the thoracic volume and air is forced out of the lungs due to the elastic recoil of lung tissues and from surface tension within the alveoli (see Fig. 10.8).

Control of breathing

The key function of the respiratory system is to provide adequate amounts of oxygen to the tissues and remove carbon dioxide. The levels of these gases in arterial blood need to remain relatively constant under a broad range of physiological circumstances. Hence the rate and depth of breathing must be carefully regulated to match physiological needs and maintain homeostasis.

Respiration is largely an involuntary act resulting from the automatic generation of rhythmic breathing by the respiratory centre in the brain stem. The respiratory centre has four parts: the inspiratory group and expiratory group in the medulla oblongata, and the pneumotaxic and apneustic centres in the pons. The integrated function of the four different groups of neurons to achieve variable rates of ventilation throughout a range of physiological needs is not completely understood.

The inspiratory group sends nerve impulses to the diaphragm and intercostals stimulating inspiration and setting the steady rate of breathing. The expiratory

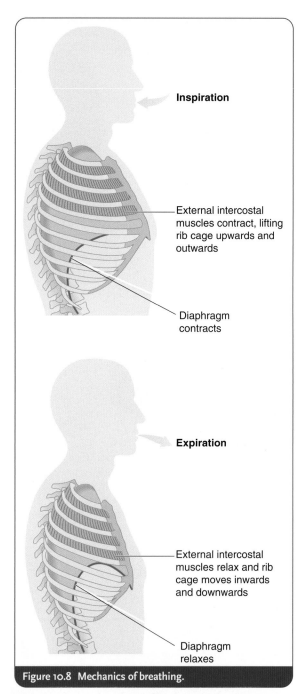

Inspiration

External intercostal muscles contract, lifting rib cage upwards and outwards

Diaphragm contracts

Expiration

External intercostal muscles relax and rib cage moves inwards and downwards

Diaphragm relaxes

Figure 10.8 Mechanics of breathing.

During inspiration the volume of the thoracic cavity increases. This results in a decrease in pressure, which causes air to flow in. During expiration the thoracic cavity resumes its relaxed position.

group is probably concerned with active expiration during laboured breathing. The pneumotaxic centre is important in regulating the duration of inspiration and the apneustic centre is responsible for sending nerve impulses that stop inspiration (Caruana-Montaldo et al 2000).

The rate and depth of breathing are controlled by homeostatic mechanisms. The homeostatic control system includes receptors, the respiratory control centre and the effectors, the diaphragm and intercostal muscles. Chemoreceptors sensitive to the concentration of carbon dioxide, hydrogen ions and oxygen are found in the medulla (central chemoreceptors) and in the aortic and carotid bodies (peripheral chemoreceptors) (Caruana-Montaldo et al 2000). Raised concentrations of carbon dioxide and hydrogen ions rather than low concentrations of oxygen usually stimulate ventilation (Blanchflower 2002).

Proprioceptors in joints are sensitive to movement and during exercise send impulses to the respiratory centre to increase ventilation and enable more oxygen to get to the contracting skeletal muscles (Caruana-Montaldo et al 2000). Many other factors influence the pattern of breathing, including hormones (Saaresranta & Polo 2002), certain drugs, alcohol, physiological circumstances such as sleep and exercise, and diseases such as asthma (Caruana-Montaldo et al 2000).

References

Balkwill F 1998 What is cancer? Biological Sciences Review 11(1):38–41

Bassett A S, Chow E W, Weksberg R, Brzustowicz L 2002 Schizophrenia and genetics: new insights. Current Psychiatry Reports 4(4):307–314

Blanchflower J 2002 Lungs and the control of breathing. Biological Sciences Review 14(4):2–5

Bowen D J 2002 Haemophilia A and haemophilia B: molecular insights. Molecular Pathology 55(2):127–144

Bozzette M 2002 Recent advances in prenatal screening and diagnosis of genetic disorders. AACN Clinical Issue 13(4):501–510

Breggin P R 1993 Toxic psychiatry. HarperCollins Publishers, London

Brock D J, Gilfillan A, Holloway S 1998 The incidence of cystic fibrosis in Scotland calculated from heterozygote frequencies. Clinical Genetics 53(1):47–49

Bulleid N J 1992 How are proteins made? Biological Sciences Review 4(5):2–4

Bulleid N J 2001 Tailor-made proteins. Biological Sciences Review 13(4):2–6

Burnet L 2003 Mechanisms of meiosis. Biological Sciences Review 15(4):20–24

Caruana-Montaldo B, Gleeson K, Zwillich W 2000 The control of breathing in clinical practice. Chest 117(1):205–225

Castronovo V, Kusaki M, Chariot A et al 1994 Homeobox genes: potential candidates for the transcriptional control of the transformed and invasive phenotype. Biochemical Pharmacology 47(1):137–143

Cattaneo E, Riganonti D, Zuccato C 2002 The enigma of Huntington's disease. Scientific American 287(6):60–65

Clark B J 1992 After a positive Guthrie – what next? Dietary management for the child with phenylketonuria. European Journal of Clinical Nutrition 46(Suppl):S33–39

Coghlan A 2000 Land of opportunity. New Scientist 168(2263): 30–33

Cohen P 1998 Clone alone. New Scientist 158(2133):32–35

Collins F S, Green E D, Guttmacher A E et al 2003 A vision for the future of genomics research. Nature 422(6934):835–847

Cookson W O C 2002 Asthma genetics. Chest 121(3) (Supplement):7S–13S

Cummings J H, Bingham S A 1998 Diet and the prevention of cancer. British Medical Journal 317(7173):1636–1640

Cunningham S, Marshall T 1998 Influence of five years of antenatal screening on the paediatric cystic fibrosis population in one region. Archives of Disease in Childhood 78(4):345–348

Dewhurst S 1998 The biological aspects of Down's syndrome. Biological Sciences Review 10(5):11–15

Doull I 2001 Recent advances in cystic fibrosis. Archives of Disease in Childhood 85(1):62–66

Gerling I C, Solomon S S, Bryer-Ash M 2003 Genomes, transcriptomes, and proteomes: molecular medicine and its impact on medical practice. Archives of Internal Medicine 163(2):190–198

Grant M 1997 Globins, genes and globinopathies. Biological Sciences Review 9(4):2–5

Gottesman I I, Shields J 1982 Schizophrenia: the epigenetic puzzle. Cambridge University Press, Cambridge

Hamilton G 1998 Let them eat dirt. New Scientist 159(2143): 26–31

Hanak J 1998 Gene therapy. Biological Sciences Review 10(4):2–5

Hecht S S 2002 Cigarette smoking and lung cancer: chemical mechanisms and approaches to prevention. Lancet Oncology 3:461–469

Itzhaki J 1999 Out of control unlocking the genetic secrets of cancer. Biological Sciences Review 11(3):36–39

Johnson B E, Cortazar P, Kelley M J 1997 The role of and significance of autocrine growth factors and neuroendocrine markers in the development of small cell lung cancer. Lung Cancer 18(Supplement 2):125–126

Jones S 1993 The language of the genes. Flamingo HarperCollins Publishers, London, p 226

Kang D 2002 Oxidative stress, DNA damage and breast cancer. AACN Clinical Issue 13(4):540–549

Kent A 1999 Patients' perspectives. In: Williams P, Clow S (eds) Genomics, healthcare and public policy. Office of Health Economics, London, p 51–57

Kendler K 2001 Twin studies of psychiatric illness: an update. Archives of General Psychiatry 58(11):1005–1014

Kiyohara C, Otsu A, Shirakawa T et al 2002 Genetic polymorphisms and lung cancer susceptibility: a review. Lung Cancer 37:241–256

Koeppen-Schomerus G, Stevenson J, Plomin R 2001 Genes and environment in asthma: a study of 4 year old twins. Archives of Disease Childhood 85(5):398–400

Kwon C, Farrell P M 2000 The magnitude and challenge of false-positive newborn screening test results. Archives of Pediatrics and Adolescent Medicine 154(7):714–718

Lawson J S, Rawlinson W D 2001 From Bittner to Barr: a viral, diet and hormone breast cancer aetiology hypothesis. Breast Cancer Research 3(2):81–85

Lehman A 1991 Keeping our genes patched up. Biological Sciences Review 4(1):12–14

Levinson D F, Holmans P, Straub R E 2000 Multicenter linkage study of schizophrenia candidate regions on chromosomes 5q, 6q, 10q and 13q. American Journal of Human Genetics 67:652–663

Lewis P, Grant M 2002 What is a gene? Biological Sciences Review 15(2):9–11

Lewis R 2003 Breast cancer: the big picture emerges. The Scientist 17(3):24–25

McLennan S 1994 The control of gene expression. Biological Sciences Review 6(5):2–5

McCormack F 1997 The structure and function of surfactant protein-A. Chest 116(6):114S–119S

McPherson K, Steel C N, Dixon J M 2000 Breast cancer – epidemiology, risk factors and genetics. British Medical Journal 321(7261):624–628

Mendelsohn E 1999 Is public policy lagging behind the science? In: Williams P, Clow S (eds) Genomics, healthcare and public policy. Office of Health Economics, London, p 64–93

Middleton L A, Peters K F 2001 Genes and inheritance. Cancer Nursing 24(5):357–369

Newman B 1999 Prenatal diagnosis. Biological Sciences Review 11(3):29–33

Nurse P 1992 The new genetics. Biological Sciences Review 5(2):15–17

O'Keefe R 2003 Transfer RNA. Biological Sciences Review 15(3):26–29

Peters J, Loud J, Dimond E et al 2001 Cancer genetics fundamentals. Cancer Nursing 24(6):446–461

Porter R 1997 The greatest benefit to mankind. HarperCollins Publishers, London

Read A 1992 Cystic fibrosis. Biological Sciences Review 4(4):18–20

Renauld J C 2001 New insights into the role of cytokines in asthma. Journal of Clinical Pathology 54(8):577–589

Rose S, Kamin L J, Lewontin R C 1984 Not in our genes. Penguin, Harmondsworth

Saaresranta T, Polo O 2002 Hormones and breathing. Chest 122(6):2165–2182

Sanders A R, Gejman P V 2001 Influential ideas and experimental progress in schizophrenia genetics research. Journal of the American Medical Association 285(22):2831–2833

Scriver C R 2002 Why mutation analysis does not always predict clinical consequences: Explanations in the era of genomics. Journal of Paediatrics 140(5):502–506

Sethi T 2002 Lung cancer. Introduction. Thorax 57(11):992–993

Simpson N, Randall R, Lenton S, Walker S 1997 Audit of neonatal screening programme for phenylketonuria and congenital hyperthyroidism. Archives of Disease in Childhood. Fetal and Neonatal Edition 77(3):F228–F234

Subramanian G, Adams M D, Venter J C, Broder S 2001 Implications of the human genome for understanding human biology and medicine. Journal of the American Medical Association 286(18):2296–2307

Susman-Shaw A, Harrington C 1999 Haemophilia: the facts. Nursing Standard 14(3):39–46

Tyfield L A 1997 Phenylketonuria in Britain: genetic analysis gives a historical perspective of the disorder but will it predict the future for affected individuals? Molecular Pathology 50(4):169–174

Venkitaraman A R 1999 Breast cancer genes and DNA repair. Science 286(5442):1100–1102

Wallis G A 1997 Getting to grips with hand development. Biological Sciences Review 10(2):33–37

Waugh A, Grant A 2001 Ross and Wilson: Anatomy and physiology in health and illness. Churchill Livingstone, Edinburgh

Wright R, Rodriguez M, Cohen S 1998 Review of psychosocial stress and asthma: an integrated biopsychosocial approach. Thorax 53(12):1066–1074

The topics and concepts introduced in the preceding chapters have been chosen to illustrate the impressive abilities and spectacular configuration of the human body. The pattern of the human body is sketched out in the beginning by the genetic legacy received from parents. The genes code for particular proteins which under the influence of time result in an unique individual reflecting the integration of heredity, environment and human experience.

The form and function of the body enables human beings to adapt to a diverse range of environments with precision and efficiency. Cells come in all shapes and sizes and, although they are described as the basic units of living matter, they are complex and extraordinary. Groups of cells form tissues of different textures and these are woven into a diverse range of organs. There is a division of labour in the body such that all organs and organ systems carry out functions that contribute to fulfilling the physiological needs of the entire body and maintaining health.

Homeostasis is synonymous with health. The concept of homeostasis helps to explain how and why we adapt to environmental change. Being healthy depends on our ability to maintain a relatively constant internal environment so that cells, tissues, organs and organ systems can function optimally. Regulation of this internal environment is achieved by hormonal and neural mechanisms that coordinate the activities within the body. A key concept in homeostasis is negative feedback in which information continuously flows between three linked components. Receptors detect changes and send signals to a controller, which integrates the information. The controller then sends instructions to effectors, which perform actions that maintain the stability of the internal environment and keep the body alive and healthy.

The food that we eat provides the raw materials for the release of energy and the building blocks for growth and development; we are literally what we eat. The molecules of life, carbohydrates, fats, proteins and nucleic acids are constructed from smaller building blocks. The same basic parts are linked together in infinite ways to produce the chemical matter of the human body. In particular, proteins play many key roles in living systems. Proteins control the movement of materials across cell membranes and therefore dictate what goes into and out of every cell in the body. Other proteins are structural and contribute to the architecture of skin, hair, muscle and the connective tissue that binds the body together. Other proteins such as enzymes and hormones have major influences on cell function.

Hormones are dynamic contributors to homeostasis and health. Hormones travel through the blood stream and when they encounter target cells that have receptors that fit their particular shape, they produce specific effects. Whilst the nervous system enables the body to adjust its processes rapidly as a consequence of changes in the environment, hormones tend to regulate more sustained processes. Hormones are potent chemicals that control growth, development, metabolism, reproduction and our ability to cope with stress.

Coordination of cell activity and the integrated functioning of organ systems by the nervous system is also achieved by chemicals. Nerve cells elicit their responses by releasing chemicals called neurotransmitters onto receiving cells. The connections between nerve cells, the synapses, play a crucial role in processing information. An important characteristic of synapses is that they can change their strength as a result of repeated use. Learning and memory depend on these changes occurring in synapses within particular parts of the brain. The number and extent of connections between neurons in the brain are changed by our experiences.

Stress is a common human experience resulting from physical, emotional, psychological or social stressors. Stress is a threat to homeostasis and to survive, the body engages in physiological and behavioural responses that enable us to adapt to stress. The stress response is designed to promote homeostasis and is coordinated by an array of chemical signals including hormones and neurotransmitters. Chronic stress is implicated in many adverse effects on health, including cardiovascular disease, mental illness, susceptibility to infections and some cancers.

The healing powers of sleep are undisputed, but much about sleep remains a mystery. Sleep contributes to health and homeostasis since it is important for our mental and physical wellbeing. The sleep–wake cycle is a good illustration of the rhythm of life in which substances, processes and activities change in a rhythmic way crucial to health. Many physiological rhythms influence or are influenced by sleep including the secretion of certain hormones, body temperature and cardiovascular functions. Some pathophysiological events or experiences also relate to the circadian phase, including pain, which may be worst at night.

Pain is a universal human experience, but the pain experience is unique to the individual. It is a multidimensional experience with physical, emotional, cognitive, social, cultural and spiritual components. Despite the suffering associated with pain there are beneficial aspects since pain warns us that something harmful is happening in our bodies. Whilst our understanding of pain mechanisms is growing the enigma of pain remains far from solved. The control of pain is complex and often illusive. Our present understanding of pain illustrates that whilst a great deal is known about the human body much more remains to be understood.

Index

Page numbers in *italic* refer to illustrations.